Reciprocal Relationships and Well-Being

This book provides a robust empirical and theoretical analysis of reciprocity and its implications for social work and social policy practices by discussing how ideas of reciprocity can be understood and applied to welfare policy and social care practices as well as how the act of reciprocity supports the well-being of citizens. Contributions from Finland, Austria, the UK, the USA and Canada illuminate the ways in which sociopolitical contexts influence the power relations between citizens, practitioners and the state, and the potential (or otherwise) for reciprocity to flourish.

This will be essential reading for social care practitioners, researchers and educationalists as well as postgraduate students in social work and related social care and community-oriented professions and social policymakers.

Maritta Törrönen is Professor of Social Work at University of Helsinki. Her main research interests concern theory of reciprocity, global welfare society, communities, power relationships, everyday life and well-being, which have points of reference with social work and social policy, childhood, child protection, family research and ethnic studies. Her recent research is linked to international social work and proactive social work. She is leading the project 'Reciprocal Encounters – Young People Leaving Care', funded by the European Union during 2016–2018.

Carol Munn-Giddings is Professor of Participative Inquiry and Collaborative Practice at Anglia Ruskin University, England. She joined Anglia Ruskin University in 1995 after many years as a social researcher and research manager in various health and social services settings. Her research focusses on ways in which citizens and citizen groups with a direct experience of a health or social situation can inform the development of appropriate health and social care services. She leads and contributes to a number of regional, national and internationally funded projects in relation to these areas and is host/mentor for the EU-funded project (2016–2018) 'Reciprocal Encounters – Young People Leaving Care', led by Professor Maritta Törrönen.

Laura Tarkiainen is a doctoral student of Social Work at University of Helsinki. Her main research interests concern discourses on prolonged unemployment, poverty and deservingness. She locates herself within the social constructionist and critical social work tradition and has a special interest in discursive methods and questions that sit on the boundary surface of social and labour market policies.

Routledge Advances in Social Work

https://www.routledge.com/Routledge-Advances-in-Social-Work/book-series/RASW

Reciprocal Relationships and Well-Being

Implications for Social Work and
Social Policy

**Edited by Maritta Törrönen, Carol
Munn-Giddings and Laura Tarkiainen**

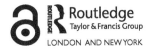
Routledge
Taylor & Francis Group
LONDON AND NEW YORK

First published 2018
by Routledge
2 Park Square, Milton Park, Abingdon, Oxon OX14 4RN

and by Routledge
711 Third Avenue, New York, NY 10017

Routledge is an imprint of the Taylor & Francis Group, an informa business

British Library Cataloguing-in-Publication Data
A catalogue record for this book is available from the British Library

Library of Congress Cataloging-in-Publication Data
A catalog record for this title has been requested

ISBN: 978-1-138-64507-3 (hbk)
ISBN: 978-0-367-43106-8 (pbk)
ISBN: 978-1-315-62836-3 (ebk)

Typeset in Times New Roman by
codeMantra

To our families

Contents

Figures and table

Figures

Table

Contributors

Antti Karisto is Emeritus Professor of Social Gerontology at the Department of Social Research, University of Helsinki. He has written extensively on health and well-being, social policy, urban topics and everyday life. More recently, he has studied the 'baby boomer' generation, retirement migration and the lifestyles of the elderly.

Bernhard Babic currently works as a researcher and lecturer at the University of Salzburg. He previously held positions in the area of research and development within national and international Non Governmental Organisations, with a special focus on social pedagogy and social work. He has also worked as an expert in external evaluation in child and youth care at the German Youth Institute (DJI). He is a board member of the Austrian Society for Social Work and a member of the interdisciplinary Human Development and Capability Association (HDCA). His latest publications are dedicated to youth and well-being research in Austria.

Thomasina Borkman, Professor of Sociology, Emerita, retired from George Mason University in Fairfax, Virginia, USA, after 32 years of teaching and research. She has specialised in research on self-help/mutual aid groups, such as groups for people who stutter and Alcoholics Anonymous, since earning her PhD from Columbia University in 1969. Her research and many of her publications are known internationally; she edited the peer-reviewed *International Journal of Self Help & Self Care* between 2007–2015. She is best known for her concept of experiential knowledge.

Claire Cameron is Professor of Social Pedagogy at University College, London (UCL) Institute of Education (IOE), where she has researched issues of care, social pedagogy, gender, the children's workforce, looked after children and early childhood education and care since the early 1990s. Currently Deputy Director of the Thomas Coram Research Unit, a specialist social science research unit at UCL IOE, and previously a social worker, she has conducted many studies, including cross-national studies, funded by the government, the EU and NGOs, of the children's

workforce and the quality of life for children in care. She is a leading figure in the introduction of social pedagogy into UK children's and adults'
workforces.

Riitta Vornanen is Professor of Social Work and the programme director
of social work studies in the Department of Social Sciences at the University of Eastern Finland. Since 2000, she has taught national specialist
postgraduate education courses for qualified (MA) social workers in the
field of social work with children, young people and families. Her main
research interests are in children's security and well-being, and social
work with children and families. Her current research interests are in
security among children and young people, processes and outcomes of
child protection, and developing intensive working models and support
services for children and families in child welfare.

Pirjo Pölkki is Professor Emerita in the Department of Social Sciences at
the University of Eastern Finland, where she worked as a Professor of
Child Welfare from 1999 to 2015. She completed her undergraduate studies and her PhD in psychology at the University of Jyväskylä. She has
worked as a researcher and senior lecturer at the University of Jyväskylä
and Kuopio, and as a clinical psychologist at Kuopio University Hospital. She has additional qualifications in child and family guidance, and
psychotherapy. Her research interests focus on preventive child care,
processes and outcomes of child protection, foster parenting and family
environment, and children's sleep. She holds several national and international positions of trust.

Tuula Heinonen is Professor with the Faculty of Social Work, University
of Manitoba. She holds a Doctorate of Philosophy from the Institute
of Development Studies, University of Sussex; a Master of Social Work
from McGill University; and an Advanced Diploma in Art Therapy from
Vancouver Art Therapy Institute. Among other research areas, her research interests include experiences of active ageing across cultural contexts, immigration and settlement among African and other newcomers,
social work in health and ageing, qualitative research methods and the
use of the arts in social work practice, research and education.

Eveliina Heino, M. Social Sciences, MA. Linguistics, Social Worker, is a
postgraduate student at the Faculty of Social Sciences, University of
Helsinki, specialising in immigration studies. For the past seven years,
she has worked as a researcher at the University of Helsinki, where her
research has focussed on social work with families, child protection, disability and unemployment. In her doctoral research, she explores how
families with a Russian background experience basic services in Finland
and construct their everyday citizenship.

Minna Veistilä, Dr of Social Sciences, Social Worker, Family Therapist, has recently defended her dissertation *From Migration to Well-being. The Construction of Social Well-being of Families with a Russian Background during Integration Processes* at the Faculty of Social Sciences, University of Helsinki. She currently works as Head of Social Services at the municipality of Sysmä, Finland. She specialises in well-being studies, and the topics of her research are related to social work with families, child protection, substance-abusing mothers and interdisciplinarity.

Niamh O'Brien is a Senior Research Fellow in the Faculty of Health, Social Care and Education at Anglia Ruskin University. Her expertise is in undertaking participatory approaches to research involving children and young people. Her interests are in research into bullying and enabling children and young people to have a voice through the research process. She is a member of the All-Party Parliamentary Group on Bullying and a Research Fellow at the Anti-Bullying Centre (ABC) at Dublin City University. Her recent doctoral thesis explored bullying at an independent day and boarding school using a Participatory Action Research approach.

Tina Moules, now retired, was formerly Director of Research in the Faculty of Health and Social Care, Anglia Ruskin University. After qualifying as a Children's Nurse, she worked in a variety of clinical areas before moving into Nurse Education at the Royal Manchester Children's Hospital and the Charles West School of Nursing, Great Ormond Street. She then moved to Anglia Ruskin University, where she was Head of Department of Children's Nursing before moving into research. She has a PhD in Health and Social Care, her thesis focussing on participatory research with children, regarding their views of hospital care.

Preface

The overall aim of the book 'Reciprocal Relationships and Well-Being: Implications for Social Work and Social Policy' is to discuss how ideas of reciprocity can be understood and applied to welfare policy and social care practices as well as how the act of reciprocity supports the well-being of citizens. In order to have a full understanding of how reciprocity and well-being can be co-created between citizens; service-users and social workers; researchers, participants and educationalists; and students, we need a thorough analysis of how experiences of reciprocity are generated in the 21st century.

In addition, we want to inspire critical discussion, offering a plurality of alternatives to individualistic approaches, focussing on interpreting the challenges of human existence from a collective perspective in communities and societies.

The primary audience for our book is social work and social care practitioners, researchers and educationalists as well as postgraduate students in social work and related social care and community-oriented professions and social policymakers.

The book will add to the current literature on social work practice, self-help and mutual aid and community development in three key ways. First, the authors are drawn from a variety of disciplines (social work, social policy, psychology, sociology, education, social pedagogy and community development), all of which welcome interdisciplinary approaches to the topic. Second, whilst focussed predominantly on the experience of Western democracies, it includes a variety of international perspectives, adding to the development of the disciplines noted. Third, it will promote innovative methodological and educational practices, which have a wider appeal to researchers and educationalists working with creative and participatory methodologies.

Importantly, we think that the topic is likely to remain relevant for the foreseeable future as discussions on reciprocal relationships remain high on political and professional agendas.

We hope you enjoy reading this book.

Maritta Törrönen, Carol Munn-Giddings and Laura Tarkiainen

Acknowledgements

The idea of this book was created during the project *Reciprocal Relationships and the Construction of Well-being during the Critical Periods of Everyday Life* (RePro), financed by the Academy of Finland for the years 2012–2016. This book was developed through the project 'Reciprocal Encounters – Young Adults Leaving Care' (ReproEncounters), which is financed by the EU in the form of a Marie Sklodowska-Curie Scholarship 2016–2018, applied for in cooperation between the University of Helsinki, Finland and Anglia Ruskin University, UK. We would like to thank the Academy of Finland for supporting the theoretical development of the concept and the empirical studies of the sub-themes. We also thank the EU for the scholarship and support, which has enabled us to widen international perspectives on theoretical and empirical considerations of reciprocity. We are thankful for the support we have received from both the University of Helsinki and Anglia Ruskin University to start and complete the book. We are grateful to you all for this opportunity.

We would also like to thank all the authors who joined the writing for this multi-year period. Half of us met each other in the European Social Work research conference in Bolzano in Italy in 2014, when we had a workshop together based on the project RePro. You were asked there if you would like to submit a chapter to a book about reciprocity. Some of you joined later. We are happy that you all joined us and have brought your invaluable contributions to the book. It has been an intensive process writing and rewriting. It has been encouraging to follow how your chapters have developed and how the concept of reciprocity has been developed so well.

Our thanks go to Dr Melanie Boyce for contributing to the ideas that shaped the content and form of the book, and her support and encouragement throughput the writing process.

We also thank our critical reviewers, Professor Richard Winter, Dr Dave Backwith, Dr Paula Sobiechowska, Professor Jeffrey Grierson and Professor Choi Won-guy, for their valuable work. The comments have undoubtedly enriched the chapters.

We want to thank Routledge and Taylor & Francis for the opportunity to publish the book for an international audience in social work and social policy. We were delighted to start the book with Emily Briggs, who worked as Editor for Science Research, Sociology, Criminology and Health and Social Care at Routledge and Taylor & Francis, and continued the work with Shannon Kneis, Claire Jarvis and Georgia Priestley. We would also like to thank Jeff Munn-Giddings for the careful editing of the chapters. For the production stage of the book we would like to thank Alexandra Andrejevich (project manager) and Erin Arata (copyeditor).

We have enjoyed editing this book, and we are happy to give it to you, our readers. We hope that you can develop the ideas of reciprocity further in your own practice.

Maritta Törrönen, Carol Munn-Giddings and Laura Tarkiainen

Introduction

In public discourse, it has been argued that since the mid-20th century, human activities have become increasingly isolated, and collectivism has diminished, particularly in Western democracies. The heightening of individualism and trends of neoliberal governance have been associated with a greater sense of insecurity, which brings along aspects of social change, including strengthened ideas of self-sufficiency in which people are increasingly obligated to take care of each other, with decreasing support from public welfare services. A counterargument to this development arises from research that demonstrates how countries with an extensive public contribution to welfare produce an improved range of well-being for their citizens compared to societies with the opposite approach. Arguments to address growing inequalities underpin the importance of looking for collective rather than individual solutions because populations identified as being most at risk of social exclusion are losing collectivist services but are less likely to meet their needs individually (Wilkinson and Pickett 2009).

However, some aspects of the neoliberal venture may inadvertently provide opportunities for rebalancing the power relations between citizens and professionals. For example, the aim to emphasise individual expertise, in its most constructive sense, may be seen as a threat to ascribed experts' authority to define human needs. Whilst this may raise objections among professionals and undermine conventional concepts of expertise, it offers the potential for experiential knowledge to be treated as expert knowledge (i.e. experts by experience of living with a health or social care situation) and considered equally alongside professional knowledge (Ruch et al. 2010). This debate may therefore encourage professionals to consider ever more carefully how they could interact with people so they feel that they have been heard.

Although the concept of reciprocity is used in a variety of disciplines, such as economics, moral philosophy, psychiatry and religious studies, as well as the social sciences – especially anthropology – sociology, psychology and social psychology, it has yet to be explored theoretically and practically in relation to its implications for social work and social policy practices. In this book, we aim to further the understanding of the concept in the social sciences in general and in social policy and social work specifically by developing a robust empirical and theoretical analysis of reciprocity. Contributing authors from different countries and areas of practice offer us a variety of ways to understand reciprocity, both in theory and in practice.

People's own interpretations of their well-being are the starting point for social work and social policy (Jordan 2007). Pierre Bourdieu (2000, p. 19) brings up an important observation on being human: 'existence humaine'. When a person seeks the meaning of life, it is of prime importance that he or she exists for others. An individual's sense of participation and their opportunities to share and participate in activities or groups that are important to them are considered to be crucial factors in human well-being. Therefore, an important aspect that underpins the book is illustrating how reciprocity is built collectively, even though an individual person is seen as a subject capable of action and agency. Through the analysis of reciprocity, we are shedding light on how most challenges, which may be discussed as the individual's problems, are, in fact, mostly connected to other people, communities and welfare systems.

The main themes and objectives

Our key aim is to illuminate collective and shared action between all the key stakeholders involved in the development and delivery of social policy and social work and social care practices as well as those doing research and educating professionals by discussing and addressing key practice themes, such as:

- What unique benefits does reciprocity offer to service users and professionals?
- What can we learn from service users' own collective actions in the community?
- Is reciprocity in general possible, given the hierarchical relationships in social work and social policy?
- Has professionalism distanced itself from the lives and experiences of service users – should practitioner and service user relationships be reframed?
  Do we need a new kind of professionalism, informed by reciprocity, something more caring?

In debating these questions, the authors will reinforce their ethos that learning from and enabling reciprocity is about enhancing and reframing social policy and social work; it is not about developing substitutes for services. Meeting the objectives will produce knowledge about how to work with and to feed reciprocity and care for one another, both informally and in the care sector.

This book embraces theoretical, empirical and discursive chapters, which at both a methodological and practical level will help in defining the goals, practices and limits to politicians' and practitioners' actions in welfare policy work and in better supporting the initiatives of service users themselves. Although the emphasis of the book is on exploring Western democracies, the authors represent different societal backgrounds, including the United Kingdom, Austria, Finland, Canada and the United States, and will draw on literature and data from a number of other countries, adding to the book varying elements of how reciprocity is understood and practised.

The book is structured into three subsections, drawing on discursive and empirical examples to illustrate the relevance of reciprocity to the development of policy and practice. We now present a summary of each section, followed by the chapter content as described by the authors:

Part I: Reciprocity: theoretical conceptualisations

The aim of this section is to reach out and to generate discussions around the concept of *reciprocity* in order to enhance our understanding of it as a potentially universally recognised phenomenon. Research into reciprocity can be seen as a contribution to international social welfare research in which the attention is focussed on well-being and the communities that hold people together (see Becker 1990, Bruni 2008, Ostrom and Walker 2003). We share the idea that the personal experience of social and societal reciprocity has profound ontological significance for an individual, and it is one of the most important factors in creating well-being. In order to have a full understanding of how well-being can be created and supported from a citizen-oriented point of view, we need a thorough theoretical analysis of how experiences of reciprocity are generated. By analysing reciprocity theoretically, we wish to clarify the meaning of collective and shared action and further develop the understanding of the concept in the social sciences, especially in social work and social policy.

Antti Karisto (Finland): Reciprocity and well-being

This chapter explores the role that social and societal reciprocity have in creating well-being. A confusing factor, however, is that there are several competing discourses on well-being in the public domain, and the significance of reciprocity varies between them. The chapter starts by discussing this conceptual confusion. Then, it clarifies the role of reciprocity in the creation of well-being by concentrating on the following topics: human relationships and everyday social intercourse, care and intergenerational relations.

Maritta Törrönen (Finland): Creating well-being through reciprocal relationships

This chapter discusses reciprocity in connection to well-being and welfare. The underlying idea suggests that reciprocal relations take place between individuals, communities and even societies. Well-being and also welfare in these relations can be depicted as dependent on how equally resources are shared, how people are respected and what kind of real possibilities people have to choose. These questions are framed by practical, symbolic and moral dimensions of reciprocity. They clarify the importance of people's social commitments and the need to transfer from individualistic services to empowerment at a community level.

Bernhard Babic (Austria): Reciprocity and normativity in social work: a complex relationship based on the Capability Approach

Starting with some basic considerations on reciprocity, this chapter reminds us of the fact that social work inevitably needs a guiding conception of what should be realised in this sphere of activity. To illustrate this in more detail, the Capability Approach and its understanding of well-being will be introduced as a normative framework, and some consequences of its operationalisation for social work will be addressed. Against this background, it becomes clear that the meaning and the informative value of reciprocity for social work cannot be assessed adequately without reflecting the respective normative orientation of this field of work.

Part II: Reciprocity in practice and community settings

This section starts by exploring the importance of reciprocal relations in groups of citizens facing similar adverse life, health or social situations. The first two chapters in this section shed some light on the core features of the reciprocal acts of both giving and receiving in group settings. The chapters will highlight the ways in which peer relationships improve and enhance group members' well-being, mobilise alternative identities and senses of normalcy, and identify distinct challenges around duty and obligation. At a wider contextual level, these chapters illustrate the importance, in social work practice and policy, of understanding and recognising the unique roles of peer relationships, groups and networks in the welfare landscape.

The next two chapters in this section focus on enablers and barriers of reciprocity in child welfare environments. Reciprocity is about mutuality and exchange, but often, social work settings, particularly in residential and family environments are characterised by hierarchical power relationships in which risk assessment predominates. A discourse of risk reinforces hierarchies of responsibility and capability, focusses on 'safety' and cuts across the central, relational role of helping people to grow and develop. The potential for reciprocity in the face of unequal power (or otherwise) is also illustrated by discussions in this section, which look at the potential for reciprocity between social workers and their service users.

Carol Munn-Giddings and Thomasina Borkman (United Kingdom and United States): Reciprocity in peer-led mutual aid groups in the community: implications for social policy and social work practices

This chapter explores one of the fastest-growing forms of community-based social support networks: mutual aid groups (MAGs) led and run by people with direct lived experience of the same health or social situations. Three unique forms of reciprocal relations are illuminated: the process of the 'sharing circle', in which peers share their experiences and listen to those of their peers; the organisational aspects of the sharing circle; and the network of specialised relationships that evolve around it. The chapter concludes with what has been learnt from this form of reciprocity and collective citizen agency.

Laura Tarkiainen (Finland): Revisions to client and professional self-categorisations during reciprocal support groups among the long-term unemployed in Finland

This chapter focusses on professionally led support groups in which alternative and revised client and professional self-categorisations may be experimented with and re-crafted. It is argued that reciprocal helping processes can mobilise alternative self-categorisations through which social work can assist its clients in reshaping and distancing themselves from culturally stigmatised categorisations used in a variety of welfare landscapes. The chapter utilises interview data from clients' and professionals' experiences in support groups that aimed to enhance the daily well-being of long-term unemployed clients in Finland. The analysis focusses on revised client and professional self-categorisations. As a result of an analysis, five categories were identified: *active life changer, supporter, equally encountered, professionally grown* and *bystander.*

Claire Cameron (United Kingdom): Risk and reciprocity in residential care: some problems with a universal norm

In this chapter, the potential for reciprocal relationships in children's residential care is discussed through analysis of interview data examining perspectives on professional-child relationships in Denmark, Flanders, Germany and England. Four types of relationship are examined before discussing the discourse of risk in residential care settings. Reciprocity, as characterised by mutual exchange as the foundation for sustaining meaningful and reparative relationships, was referred to less often than more instrumental purposes of relationships. The articulation of risk and risk assessments acted as a further barrier to developing reciprocity in the responses from English residential care homes. Axel Honneth's (1995) concept of recognition, as extended to include young people's participation, is suggested as a more promising way forward than reciprocity for conceptualising relationships in residential care.

Riitta Vornanen and Pirjo Pölkki (Finland): Reciprocity and relationship-based approach in child welfare

Reciprocity as a concept has not been widely discussed in child welfare research. This chapter concentrates on reciprocity from the perspective of a relationship-based approach. Reciprocity may offer a way to understand and focus on the relationships, engagement and power between the social worker, the parents and the children. The core of the concept is in the nature and quality of the relationships between the parents and their children. Social workers may need to intervene in these sensitive and private family relationships, and the foundation of the work rests on how these relationships are understood. The developmental origins of reciprocity need to be known in order to understand children's growth relative to the reciprocal and secure relationships. Child welfare social work entails working with and within relationships. The concept of reciprocity strengthens the understanding of the meaning of relations and the importance of belonging and recognition in child welfare.

Part III: Reciprocity: methodological and educational issues

The final section explores the importance of reciprocity and complementary participatory methods in both research and educational practices – activities that underpin the development of social work policy and practices. The chapters highlight how the integration of bidirectionality, mutual caring, reciprocity and meaningful relationships into social work can contribute to effective and reflective methods. The chapters in this section cover a range of settings and issues that, again, tackle the potential for reciprocity in seemingly hierarchical relations between researchers and the people they research; between co-researcher teams involving adults, children and young people; and between graduate social work students and their advisors in contexts in which rigour, indicators of individual achievement and evaluation of outcomes prevail.

Tuula Heinonen (Canada): Reciprocity with graduate students fostered through creativity

This chapter focusses on reciprocity in graduate student-advisor relationships that occur in a context of academic guidance and mentorship introduced through a reflexive, shared process. Nicola Simmons and Shauna Daley (2013), who view the creative process as the highest level of thinking, provided the impetus for an introduction of a mixed media exercise in which students created drawings and short narratives to express their impressions about their year's works. In return, the author produced for students a response art piece (Fish 2008), which led to shared insights and more effective and enhanced advisor-student relationships.

Eveliina Heino and Minna Veistilä (Finland): Narrative reflection as a reciprocal method

This chapter focusses on the reciprocal elements of narrative reflection in interview-based research. The authors define reciprocal elements as parts of narrative reflection that promote feelings of fair treatment between researchers and interviewees. The study data consist of 25 initial and 9 follow-up interviews among families with a Russian background living in Finland. The analysis focusses on the structure of the interviews and the interactions between researchers and interviewees. As a result of this study, three reciprocal elements are identified: *creating a shared understanding, participation* and *recognition*.

Niamh O´Brien, Tina Moules and Carol Munn-Giddings (United Kingdom): Negotiating the research space between young people and adults in a PAR study exploring school bullying

This chapter explores the process of evaluating the individual and collective view of participation in a Participatory Action Research (PAR) project carried out by an adult researcher and five young researchers. The PAR framework allowed for a commitment to continuous information sharing, reflection and action. The process of evaluating participation on three occasions empowered the team to reflect on the reciprocal relationships that developed between the adult and the young researchers. The study acknowledges participation as fluid and dynamic. Furthermore, recognising that power can be shared between adult and young researchers is crucial to the development of reciprocal relationships in research.

References

Becker, L. C., 1990. *Reciprocity.* London: Routledge & Kegan Paul.

Bourdieu, P., 2000. *Pascalian Meditations.* Stanford: Stanford University Press.

Bruni, L., 2008. *Reciprocity, Altruism and the Civil Society. In Praise of Heterogeneity.* London and New York: Routledge.

Fish, B., 2008. Formative Evaluation Research of Arts-Based Supervision in Art Therapy Training. *Journal of the Art Therapy Association*, 25 (2), 70–77.

Honneth, A. 1995. *The Struggle for Recognition: The Moral Grammar of Social Conflicts.* Cambridge: Polity Press.

Jordan, B., 2007. *Social Work and Wellbeing.* Dorset: Russell House Publishing.

Ostrom, E., and Walker, J., 2003. *Trust and Reciprocity. Interdisciplinary Lessons from Experimental Research.* New York: Russel Sage Foundation.

Ruch, G., Turney, D., and Ward, A., 2010. *Relationship-Based Social Work: Getting to the Heart of Practice.* London: Jessica Kingsley.

Simmons, N., and Daley, S., 2013. The Art of Thinking: Using Collage to Stimulate Scholarly Work. *Canadian Journal of the Scholarship of Teaching and Learning*, 4 (1), 1–11.

Wilkinson, R., and Pickett, K., 2009. *The Spirit Level: Why More Equal Societies Almost Always Do Better.* London: Allen Lane.

Part I

Reciprocity

Theoretical conceptualisations

1 Reciprocity and well-being

Antti Karisto

Introduction

[E]ach gift is part of a system of reciprocity in which the honours of giver and recipient are engaged. It is a total system in that every item of status or of spiritual or material possession is implicated for everyone in the whole community. The system is quite simple: just the rule that every gift has to be returned in some specified way sets up a perceptual cycle of exchanges within and between generations. In some cases the specified return is of equal value, producing a stable system of statuses; in others it must exceed the value of the earlier gift, producing an escalating contest of honour. The whole society can be described by the catalogue of transfers that map all the obligations between its members. The cycling gift system is the society.

(Douglas 1990, viii–ix)

The quote above by Mary Douglas reflects the ethos of the present chapter, in which I explore the essence of reciprocity from the viewpoint of well-being. Let me, however, begin by recollecting a personal memory that led me to consider the theme. A quarter of a century ago, I visited the School for Advanced Urban Studies, which operates under the auspices of the University of Bristol. At the end of the week, the researchers had the habit of going down to the pub. The evening proceeded in such a way that one would offer a round to everyone, and then it would be the turn of the next. There were around ten of us, and I became restless when I thought about when it would be my turn. Why on earth should I offer drinks to such a large group of people, most of whom I hardly knew? Perhaps I would buy a round next Friday or the Friday after. Or should I offer to buy it now to avoid being labelled a freeloader and risk losing face?

I decided to raise the topic of buying rounds, and the rules of the game were explained to me. Naturally, no record was kept of who had bought what; you simply trusted that everyone would commit, more or less, to the principle of reciprocity. If one Friday night did turn out to be expensive, you got to drink for free on many following Fridays, and in the long run, everything would work out fair and square. As a temporary guest, I wasn't expected to buy a round, but these urban sociologists in the pub were extremely surprised at my description of Finnish pub culture, where everyone buys their own drinks, or, if not, they settle up during the same night.

My pub experience gave me food for thought; it forced me to ponder offering and reciprocity. Offering can be an empty word; reciprocity can be spurious. If accounts are immediately settled, then the bother of paying is just passed from one person to another, in turn. With mechanical reciprocity, the boozing continues, but the kind of reciprocity that really sweetens life seems to require something else: disinterested willingness to give, spontaneous broad-mindedness, tactful understanding of the situation and appreciation of the nature of the good life.

In this chapter, I investigate reciprocity and its importance in the creation of well-being. I begin by making a few observations about cultural variation in everyday social intercourse and then move on to the level of concepts. If reciprocity is a difficult notion open to many interpretations, then so is well-being. A confusing factor is that there are several competing discourses on well-being, and the significance of reciprocity varies between them. I will give particular thought to well-being in human relationships as reciprocity is connected to them almost by definition. I will also examine the kind of 'general reciprocity' that occurs in social policy and social work. Finally, I investigate reciprocity in old age and in intergenerational relations. When we are old, we are particularly dependent on one another, and the sustainability of our well-being requires a 'generationally intelligent' social policy.

Culturally defined forms of reciprocity

As a Finn, I am accustomed to the exchange of words in everyday comings and goings being rather terse. In his novel, Hannu Raittila presents this in an indisputable way:

> In speech in foreign languages a Finn is always disturbed by the fact that sentences have all kinds of unnecessary phrases and politeness forms. They make the language difficult and awkward to speak and obscure its meaning. In Finnish, the matter is said in the simplest and most unambiguous way possible, and then we wait to see what the other replies. If there is nothing to say, we are silent.
>
> (Raittila 2001, p. 40)

We are often silent. Linguists have characterised reticence and 'minimal politeness' as being typical of Finns. We react to open rudeness, but we do not expect language to be particularly polite (e.g. Jaakkola 2008, pp. 113–115). Does Finland suffer from a particular deficit of politeness and respect of the kind that Richard Sennett (2003) considers to be a unifying feature of modern societies? Finns are certainly capable of saying 'thank you', but one symptom of the paucity of explicitly polite reciprocity that is embedded in the Finnish language or mind is our lack of an equivalent for the useful word 'please'. Well, of course, we have the phrasal equivalents *ole hyvä* and *olkaa hyvä* (literally 'be good'), but using them is already something of an effort: You need to use two words and choose between the formal and informal form of address. Perhaps for this reason, these words are used far less than quickly delivered words in many other languages (Karisto 2010, pp. 74–77). In Finnish, *kiitos* ('thank you') is like a full stop. You can reply to it with *eipä kestä* ('no problem') or the more ceremonious *kiitos on minun puolellani* ('my pleasure'; literally, 'the gratitude is on my side'), but those phrases have the same tone: That's enough thanking! Obligatory phrases are recited, but reciprocity is not expected to continue over and above this point.

Finland is considered a *low context* culture in which people typically attempt to produce so-called *first-level* descriptions. Things are said 'the way they are'; the relationship between speech and its subject is considered unambiguous. This contrasts with *second-level* descriptions or *high context* cultures in which speech does not refer so much to reality as to other speech concerning that reality (Daun 1989, Baudrillard 1991, see Alapuro 1997, pp. 184–186).

The division between low or high contexts or first and second levels is, of course, a generalising typology that may exaggerate cultural differences. There is no reason to consider a paucity of reciprocity to be an essential characteristic of Finnish culture or brand Finnish manners as shoddier or coarser than those of other cultures. While in other cultures, politeness is cultivated more intensely, social interaction is not necessarily more warm-hearted. It is unlikely that Brits are always as thoroughly broad-minded and generous as they implied in that Bristol pub. And perhaps it is an example of 'orientalism' (Said 2011) to think that reciprocity is always the spice of life in Eastern cultures. For example, benevolence and sympathy (*amae*) are said to be at the centre of the Japanese way of life. Gifts are given in many situations, for instance, when a colleague's daughter gets married, irrespective of whether one personally knows the individual concerned or not. A gift is always followed by a reciprocal gift, but the exchange of gifts is normatively regulated and carefully apportioned. A reciprocal gift cannot be too modest or too extravagant; in some situations, it must be a defined fraction of the value of the gift received. This even obliges people to keep a written record of the gifts they have received and discover their monetary value (Davies and Ikeno 2002, pp. 238–239). But doesn't norm-driven, carefully calculated reciprocity feel more like an obligation than real reciprocity (see also Becker 1986, pp. 73–74)?

Forms of reciprocity are culturally specific, and it is difficult to place them in rank order. Forms of reciprocity are also malleable. In recent years, there has been a greater abundance of Finnish phrases and expressions; linguistic reciprocity has clearly become richer. The new generation of service sector workers draws its influences from practices abroad, and presumably people in Finnish pubs also behave differently from my generation in its youth.

Organic reciprocity, not a mechanistic exchange

The kind of reciprocity that boosts well-being does not need to be of the expressive, effusive kind; rather, it can also be realised in a restrained Finnish way, without melodrama. Nonetheless, in some way, it must be flexible and organic. Reciprocity includes giving, even if we do not immediately receive something in return. Reciprocity can only be realised over the course of time, and it does not always need to occur. It can be more of a disposition: a general willingness to do good for others. For example, the core of friendship is just this willingness. We have friends, so we can turn to them, even if we don't actually turn to them, and although they cannot always help. The modern understanding of friendship, in contrast, is freedom from binding obligations (Pahl 2000, p. 37). Hospitality is another model for reciprocity and searching for a good life. For example, the sharing of meals is meant to be continual. The pattern 'give, receive, give in return...' identifies an open-ended process in which some imbalance is always present (Boisvert and Heldke 2016, p. 51).

In reciprocity that occurs in social interaction, there must be space for situational sensitivity (Naukkarinen 2011). Spontaneity and surprise are good – there is little enjoyment in getting something one was already certain of receiving. It feels much better to receive something unexpectedly and from an unlikely source.

Nonetheless, an entirely predictable, mechanistic exchange, or what Serge-Christophe Kolm (2000a, p. 14) terms 'self-sustained sequential exchange', also has its uses. It is better that norms oblige us to perform friendly gestures rather than entice us to engage in misanthropy. Even mechanical or superficial reciprocity maintains a sense of community, and neglecting it can be fatal in the same way that open arrogance is. However, mechanical reciprocity is hardly a bottomless wellspring of well-being, and neither is simply refraining from impoliteness. Well-being is something more than a lack of problems and grievances or their successful regulation – contrary to common thinking in social policy and social work, where *well-being* and *welfare* are often conflated. In Finnish, there is also confusion due to the fact that the word *hyvinvointi* is used to describe the good life of an individual (*well-being*), the good produced by the welfare state (*welfare*) and any form of indulgent and momentary gratification (*wellness*). Even actual well-being has many forms, and the Finnish sociologist Erik Allardt (1976), for example, divides it into three broad dimensions: *Having, Loving* and *Being*.

The many forms of well-being

Not all forms of reciprocity are good as reciprocity can also involve revenge for ill treatment. However, my focus here is on reciprocity that is beneficial in one way or other – but beneficial for what? Well-being, like reciprocity, is a multifaceted and slippery concept. Although the nature of the good life has been pondered for millennia and the multiplicity of well-being has often been emphasised, in public discourse, it is basically understood as *Having*, i.e. the material goods that a person possesses. In publicity, well-being is embedded in the economy. It is believed that well-being is produced when the economy is left to function free from interference. The well-being of the economy is an issue of absolute primacy because it is considered to trickle down to create individual well-being.

Even if the economic approach to well-being has become dominant, it is by no means the only perspective. There are several competing discourses on well-being, and the significance of reciprocity varies between them. For promoters of health, well-being, above all, means a healthy and well-functioning body. In social policy, it is the good produced by the welfare state, the regulation of poverty and other problems – at bottom, security. From an ecological perspective, sustainability is the crucial precondition of well-being. It may mean transcendental or aesthetic peak experiences and so on. Well-being is much discussed, but one person understands it one way and the next in a different way. Politicians and other actors are quick to appeal to well-being because it is the magic word that also seems to legitimise the pursuit of their particular interests (Karisto 2010, pp. 15–19).

Reciprocity has been highly prominent in economic notions of well-being (e.g. Gérard-Varet *et al.* 2000, Gintis 2000a, 2000b). In fact, it has been economists who have developed the formal theory of reciprocity – game theory – the furthest. In particular, the theme of reciprocity has been cultivated in discussions on alternatives to a pure market economy: caring economy, social enterprises and corporate social responsibility, women's banks and microcredit and finance, fair trade practices and time banking, in which the transfer of services does not involve the exchange of money but the exchange of time and services provided for others (Bruni 2008, Koskiaho 2014, Hirvilammi 2015).

Nevertheless, reciprocity has been even more widely discussed in the social sciences, psychology, anthropology and moral philosophy. In these disciplines, reciprocity and economic exchange are considered two different, even mutually exclusive, principles of exchange (Polanyi 2001, p. 47, Kujala and Danielsbacka 2015, pp. 20–21 and 39–43). For example, the Swedish sociologist Sten Johansson has warned about mixing the rules of private and economic life, terming it 'prostitution', the confusing of political and economic spheres 'corruption' and the intermingling of political and private life 'nepotism' (Johansson 1979, pp. 101–103). According to Niklas Luhmann, social subsystems – the economy, politics, the welfare state, science, art, the media and others – are 'autopoietic', i.e. self-referential. There is interaction between them, but each has its own way of communicating, its own 'medium' and its own 'code' (Jalava and Kangas 2013). Things turn out badly if the medium of one subsystem becomes dominant in the other subsystems, with corruption and prostitution being among the consequences when 'money talks'.

Loving, of course, is closer to reciprocity than the other dimensions of well-being distinguished by Allardt (1976). Some level of reciprocity is an absolute precondition for well-being based on human relations. The kind of partnership or friendship where flows of support and emotion only travel in one direction is doomed to fail. The social exchange that occurs among family and friends is sometimes considered the only genuine form of reciprocity (see Kolm 2000a, p. 28, Bruni 2008, p. xii). Perceived well-being is strongly affected by the reciprocity that occurs in social interaction: whether we receive love and whether we give it, and how we value and treat one another. In people's own interpretations of their well-being, human relationships, alongside health, are considered the most significant factors (e.g. Haapola *et al.* 2013, p. 84).

Well-being accumulates in different ways in its different dimensions. While hankering after *Having*, it might feel that well-being grows at the expense of others as there is only a certain amount of material goods to be divided at any one time. Well-being built on human relationships, in contrast, does not diminish, even if it is given to others. On the contrary, those who enjoy the greatest well-being are those for whom goodwill and care for the well-being of their nearest and dearest are important (Sortheix 2014).

The various dimensions of well-being relate differently not only to reciprocity but to one another. For example, poor health is a *corrosive disadvantage* (Wolff and De-Shalit 2007) as when health is lost, other forms of well-being threaten to vanish. Nonetheless, even if a person is in perfect health, this will not necessarily increase her other forms of well-being. In contrast, good human relationships and reciprocity are thought to have a *fertile functioning*, i.e. a particular ability to promote other forms of well-being (*ibid.*) and to prevent them from being negatively impacted by various kinds of loss. According to Alvin W. Gouldner (1960), reciprocity may also initiate social cooperation in the early phases of group consolidation, in which others are easily viewed with suspicion, e.g. in interaction between immigrants and nationals (Manatschal 2015, p. 243).

Demanding reciprocity

Alongside warm interpersonal emotions, cool intellect is also reciprocal. According to the Swedish essayist Horace Engdahl (2013, p. 33), the criteria for intelligence lie 'not in the ability to say profound things but in the ability to listen. Intelligence requires two brains, their interplay'.

It is through reciprocity that we find our place in the world (Thompson 2013, p. 39). Our identities are constructed on the basis of our social interactions with others and our abilities to see the world through others' eyes. 'Through the thou a person becomes I', wrote Martin Buber (1999, p. 52). Similarly, Emmanuel Levinas reminds us that being true to ourselves includes having a sense of responsibility towards others (see Sennett 1999, p. 145).

Reciprocity is good for both the individual and the community. It reinforces human relationships, increases trust and expands cultural and social capital. Nevertheless, it is not an automatic dispenser of happiness. Martha Nussbaum (2001, see Bruni 2008, pp. 8–9) has emphasised the enormous significance of friendship, love and other *relational goods* but has also spoken of their fragility. Reciprocity in human relations is never certain. On the contrary, well-being connected to human relationships is unstable, and virtuous circles built on reciprocity are easily broken. According to Fransesco Alberoni (1989), nothing beyond the new relationship seems to have space in the consciousness of someone who has fallen in love, and this source of well-being feels completely inexhaustible. Nevertheless, the rapture produced by being in love is generally just momentary ecstasy, and the hubris of well-being can be followed by its nemesis. If all goes well, the lovers' tumultuous emotions coalesce into life-affirming prosaic love, but for the less fortunate, love evaporates and even becomes its opposite: hate.

The problem with well-being based on *Having* is that we are never satisfied. A successful purchase only brings a momentary glow; there never seems to be enough material well-being. However, a similar kind of 'pursuit of the unattainable' (Ehrnrooth 1995) also features in reciprocity. Such high demands are placed upon it that we can never entirely realise them.

In the ethics of reciprocity, a famous ideal type is *agápe*: pure altruistic love – i.e. the kind that is 'patient and kind, does not envy or boast, is not arrogant or rude, does not insist on its own way, is not irritable or resentful, and does not rejoice at wrongdoing'. However, this kind of love, which 'bears all things, believes all things, hopes all things, and endures all things', seems to be above and beyond the kind of reciprocity found in everyday life (Bruni 2008, p. 50). 'Do unto others as you would have them do unto you' is the golden rule of ethics, but in practice, we never realise this in its entirety. Nonetheless, the mighty precept is necessary. Although (or precisely because) we are forced to live our everyday lives in the framework of factual necessities, moral guidelines and 'the principle of hope' have their purposes (e.g. Ehrnrooth 2014). 'Pursuit of the unattainable', the attempt to reach beyond actual reality, is said to be a characteristic striving of people living in the Western world (Ehrnrooth 1995, pp. 34–50), but the golden rule of ethics and its variations are certainly recognised in other cultures (e.g. Thompson 2013, p. 45). This is also proof of the universal value of reciprocity.

In moral philosophy, there are numerous variants of the golden rule. Immanuel Kant's *categorical imperative* obliges us to place ourselves in another person's shoes and act in such a way that our actions could become a universal law. *The face* was the central metaphor used by Levinas (1996) when writing about encountering another person. When we look another person – even a stranger – in the face, we should be ready to take responsibility for that person. Buber's (1999) comparable ethical imperative was *Thou*, which is entirely different to the *It* of objectified human relationships. According to Buber, we should live in the world of Thou and cherish the

I–Thou relationship so that the goal of altruistic reciprocity is realised: 'between the I and the Thou there is no striving, no demands nor anticipation' (*ibid.*, p. 34).

Ethical ideals linked to reciprocity are a kind of compass for well-being: They give us the direction in which to strive and perhaps also the power to do so. Raymond D. Boisvert and Lisa Heldke (2016, pp. 59–65) appoint Jane Addams, a pioneer of social work, as an 'inspirational individual' who kept alive the sense of reciprocal dependence. Three ethical principles were adopted in Hull House, a neighbourhood settlement for immigrants that was founded by Addams: 'to teach by example, to practice cooperation, and to practice social democracy, that is, egalitarian, or democratic, social relations across class lines' (Knight 2005, p. 182). In practice, Hull House offered a comprehensive set of social services and cultural, recreational and educational activities for people who could hardly be more different from the people with whom Addams herself grew up (Boisvert and Heldke 2016, p. 63).

The limitations of reciprocity

Sociology and anthropology have focussed more on describing the practical forms of reciprocity and solidarity that appear in communal life than on their ethical requirements or content in an ideal world. It is comforting to note that in practice, people do not always think only of their immediate benefits. Empathy, generosity and offering, in other words reciprocity, are found in every society – even in modern society, where it is feared that the individual, in pursuit of personal gain, will trample others under foot in an atmosphere of heightened individualism.

Nonetheless, according to Marcel Mauss (1999), a gift is not given without an expectation that the giver will receive a gift in return. We compete even in munificence; even a debt of gratitude is a debt. In the closest human relationships, interaction can still be directed by altruistic benevolence in which help is given, even at the expense of the well-being of the helper. Outside such relationships, a precondition for giving is nevertheless that it is worthwhile or cost-effective. Expressed in plain technical terms, helping is worthwhile if the cost is 'smaller than the benefit of the expected return service times the probability of receiving that service' (Danielsbacka 2013, p. 31).

According to evolutionary psychologists, the desire to help is genetically encoded within us, but it is more likely to be directed towards those who are close to us. How far the *circle of empathy* extends in practice is dependent on the cultural environment (Pinker 2011, p. 668, Danielsbacka 2013, p. 30). It usually includes family members, who receive help almost unconditionally. In contrast, helping friends is already bound up with the quality of each individual relationship and the general norms that govern friendships. Altruistic giving is, after all, the exception, but so is the exclusive pursuit of personal gain; most commonly, we operate between these two extremes (Kolm 2000b, p. 115).

Nowhere does the circle of empathy extend limitlessly. It covers 'us' but not 'them' or 'others'. It is no wonder that Sennett (1999, pp. 136–139) considers the pronoun 'we' to be so dangerous. By cultivating it, we strengthen our circles of empathy and build their internal senses of community, but the word 'us' is also swiftly repeated when excluding 'others'. If empathy and reciprocity are genetically programmed, then so is the binary opposition of 'us' and 'them', and this opposition can be reproduced in the name of 'us'.

When discussing 'the corrosion of character', Sennett (1999) claims that reciprocity is weakened by societal changes. Under the conditions of new neoliberal capitalism, people are forced to adopt an individualistic 'flexibility', and reciprocal loyalty is no longer the self-evident foundation of communal life. According to Sennett, a character that is incapable of empathy will become more common. This has also been discussed by Christopher Lasch (1979) in his analysis of the *culture of narcissism* and was detailed decades before by Georg Simmel (1903/2005, pp. 33–36) in his description of the reserved habitus of people raised in modern urban society. In the metropolis, it is simply impossible to encounter others as whole personalities. One cannot look them in the face, cannot become involved in all their possible woes and troubles – not without finding oneself in a 'completely unbearable spiritual state', at least (*ibid.*, p. 35). We learn to pass others by.

The dominant form of solidarity in modern society is said to be *negative solidarity*, which is demonstrated by not interfering in the business of others (Kortteinen 1982, pp. 251–252). That, too, is solidarity, and a certain form of reciprocity, as we do not expect others to interfere in our affairs either. Although non-interference and the reciprocal guarding of each other's privacy are a necessity of sorts and sometimes even an indication of tact, nonetheless, they should not be turned into a virtue. On the contrary, negative solidarity easily leads us to view 'others' as simply not being there at all: We do not harm them, but nor do we respect them; they are simply ignored. Those on the fringes, or outside, of the circle of empathy go unnoticed and are easily abandoned. Simmel was conscious of this when writing about how aloofness or indifference towards others – which he also considered to be a guarantee of personal freedom – can, in an instant, 'break into hatred and fight' (Simmel 2005, p. 35). Buber crystallises the relationship between positive and negative solidarity by stating that a person must live in the world of *It* but 'he who lives with *It* alone is not a man' (Buber 1999, p. 34).

Welfare state reciprocity

In recent times, increasing calls have been made for people to take greater care of one another rather than leaving this care to the welfare state. It is nevertheless unrealistic to imagine that in families and local communities, entirely untapped reciprocal resources lie dormant, as is claimed by those supporting individual solutions or advocating for 'implicit familialism' (Leitner 2003). Because the circle of moral responsibility does not necessarily extend very far, not everything can rest on individual behaviour. If we cannot look 'others' in the face, their needs can be addressed through social policy and social work. Reciprocity that produces well-being is not only interaction between individuals; rather, social life and social policy are 'fundamentally a question of reciprocity' (Kolm 2000a, p. 16, Bruni 2008, pp. ix–xii).

Richard Titmuss's (1970) famous example of *general* or *indirect reciprocity* was that of giving blood. Blood donors do not expect payment or any other immediate gift in return. They do not even know who will receive the blood they have donated – just as they do not know the purpose for which their individual tax payments will be used. Blood donors and taxpayers simply trust that reciprocity will occur: Tax revenue will also be used for their benefit, and they will be given blood if they happen to need it.

Jyri Liukko, a Finnish researcher of social policy, has dubbed social insurance to be a 'solidarity machine'. Social insurance is a moral technology that makes solidarity automatic, and which 'is always in some way linked to collaborative action and reciprocity' (Liukko 2013, p. 8). Similarly, the entire welfare state can be considered an institution that is based on and realises general reciprocity.

General reciprocity, however, is not symmetrical in the same way as genuine reciprocity between individuals might be. One does not receive services and income transfers that are directly equated to one's tax contributions. Means testing results in help being given to those who need it the most. Social support differs from true reciprocity in terms of its redistributive nature, but it can also be understood as 'delayed reciprocity' or as investment. In the long run, society enjoys a return on its investment, and the public good accumulates. Social investments nevertheless require time; the return may be long in coming, and sometimes, there is no payback for the help provided. For this reason, too, the public sector is better suited to making social investments and engaging in general reciprocity than are private actors (Sipilä 2011, p. 363).

Reciprocity in old age and in intergenerational relationships

In general, there is no need to understand reciprocity solely as one giving something to another, who, in turn, gives something of equal worth in return. For example, intergenerational reciprocity is often based on 'chains'. A gives to B and B, in turn, gives to C (Kolm 2000a, p. 7, Kolm 2008, pp. 16, 46 and 79). The older generation pays for the younger generation's schooling, and the latter pays for the education of the next. An example of a chain in the other direction, and of general reciprocity, is pension policy. In pay-as-you-go pension systems, the lion's share of workers' pension contributions is used to pay the pensions of those already retired, and the workers must trust that this practice will continue in the future, when they too have retired.

Taking care of one's own children is a universally internalised obligation. In many countries, the interests of children are also enshrined in law, and if parents seriously neglect these interests, then their parenthood can be limited. In contrast, in Finland, there are no statutory obligations to care for one's parents, but, of course, there are normative obligations. From the perspective of their well-being, it is important that the elderly receive the care they need and can also otherwise interact with members of the younger generation. Intergenerational social intercourse is important to the elderly (Bengtson 2001), but young people also desire it, at the latest when they become old themselves and want to maintain contact with their own children and grandchildren.

For elderly people, reciprocity is a particularly central source of well-being; without it, it is futile to speak of *successful ageing*. Elderly people typically expect that others will have the time for social intercourse, and this concerns both intimate relationships and professional care. Of course, a professional carer also gains a sense of pleasure from having the time to properly encounter others as whole human beings rather than as the latest home help customers of the day. However, for professional carers, time is often short. Care work is organised in the same way as other forms of production, and this prevents the deepening of reciprocity. A conflict arises between 'doing and encountering' (Palomäki and Toikko 2007).

In spite of its apparent asymmetry, care is also essentially reciprocal. Care is about concern for others and taking responsibility, looking after others and carrying their cares (Fisher and Tronto 1990). It is a relational activity, based on mutual dependency (Martela 2012), whose telos is restoring the autonomy of the care receiver (De Lange 2011). Care requires reciprocal tact, adapting oneself to the pace and rhythm of the other (see Naukkarinen 2011). For example, in family care, the reciprocal functions of the provider and the recipient of care complement each other so subtly that it is sometimes impossible to distinguish the role of the carer from that of the recipient (Andersson 2007). Nevertheless, there is often a divide between these roles; for example, someone suffering from severe dementia can be entirely at the mercy of others. The abilities to engage in reciprocity and accept responsibility are particularly tested when the other person no longer seems to be an autonomous agent nor appears capable of giving anything.

Bryan S. Turner (1989, Pilcher 1995, p 105) sees the precarious social status of the elderly as resulting from their often being solely recipients of care and help when their abilities to give and to engage in immediate reciprocity have diminished. This can be fateful in a society where 'the ideology of social parasitism' prevails, and helplessness is a sign of weakness and dependence on others a mark of shame (Sennett 1999, p. 139–140). When we have started to measure the 'success' of old age against the ideal of *productive ageing*, in which the greatest value is given to work and work-like activities, we no longer understand that those who have become helpless and unfit for work also have, and particularly have had, something to give.

Jari Pirhonen (2015), who has adapted Charles Taylor's (1992) and Axel Honneth's (2005) *recognition theory* to eldercare in Finland, is concerned that the humanity of incapacitated elderly people will be lost in their 'patienthood' or 'customership'. Indeed, this will happen if the elderly are seen merely as clients, patients or medical cases rather than as whole human beings and unique biographical creatures. A new kind of professionalism, informed by theories of reciprocity and well-being, is also needed in eldercare. This professionalism is 'generationally intelligent' (Biggs and Lowenstein 2011) when it is sensitive to the life-courses and lifeworlds of 'clients' who belong to different generations than their carers.

Our thinking about old age is far too polarised, placed either in a framework of choices or a framework of necessities. Incapacity and dependence on others seem completely incompatible with activeness and autonomy, which are nowadays so strongly emphasised (Kröger *et al.* 2007, pp. 11–13). In old age, agency and activeness are important, but they are often understood only narrowly, through rationalistic choices and in terms of productive activities (Grenier and Phillipson 2013). Referring to Alasdair MacIntyre (1999, pp. 1–9), Pirhonen (2015) writes that

> humanity is not defined by rationality and self-determination, but by biology, frailty and dependence. We are born completely dependent, we create the illusion of self-determination during our adulthood and we are forced to recognise our dependence once more as our capacity declines with aging.

Simon Biggs and Ariela Lowenstein (2011) call for *generational intelligence*, a form of reflexive reciprocity, in both private and public life. They advocate that our perspectives should not be defined simply by the typical aims of our own age groups and generations and our own immediate benefits and desires. We should remember the existence of other generations and understand that they too have legitimate interests, which are balanced with our own in social policies.

It is particularly difficult for us to empathise with those generations yet to be born. Nevertheless, we must do this (Kolm 2000a, p. 29) as it is a requirement of the social sustainability of well-being. The state of the world should be at least as good when we leave it as when we were born into it (Becker 1980, p. 228). We must also offer something to future generations, and we cannot ask them to pick up our tab just because they won't have a chance to buy us a round.

References

Alapuro, R., 1997. *Suomen älymystö Venäjän varjossa.* Helsinki: Tammi.
Alberoni, F., 1989. *Rakastuminen.* Helsinki: Otava. (Original: Innamoramento e amore. Milano: Aldo Garzanti Editore, 1979.)

Allardt, E., 1976. *Hyvinvoinnin ulottuvuudet.* Helsinki: WSOY.

Andersson, S., 2007. *Kahdestaan kotona – tutkimus vanhoista pariskunnist*a. Helsinki: Stakes, tutkimuksia 169.

Baudrillard, J., 1991. *Amerikka.* Helsinki: Loki-kirjat. (Original: Amérique. Paris: Editions Grasset & Fasquelle, 1986.)

Becker, L. C., 1986. *Reciprocity.* London and New York: Routledge & Kegan Paul.

Bengtson, V. L., 2001. Beyond the Nuclear Family: The Increasing Importance of Multigenerational Bonds. *Journal of Marriage and Family* 63(1):1–16.

Biggs, S., and Lowenstein, A., 2011. *Generational Intelligence. A Critical Approach to Age Relations.* London: Routledge.

Boisvert, R. A., and Heldke, L., 2016. *Philosophers at Table. On Food and Being Human.* London: Reaktion Books.

Bruni, L., 2008. *Reciprocity, Altruism and the Civil Society. In Praise of Heterogeneity.* London: Routledge.

Buber, M., 1999. *Minä ja Sinä.* Helsinki: WSOY. (Original: Ich und Du. Leipzig: Insel-Verlag, 1923.)

Danielsbacka, M., 2013. *Vankien vartijat. Ihmislajin psykologia, neuvostosotavangit ja Suomi 1941–1944.* Historiallisia tutkimuksia Helsingin yliopistosta XXXII. Helsinki: Helsingin yliopiston filosofian, historian, kulttuurin ja taiteiden tutkimuksen laitos.

Daun, Å., 1989. *Svensk mentalitet.* Stockholm: Nordsteds Akademiska Förlag.

Davies, R. J., and Ikeno, O., 2002. The Japanese Mind. Understanding the Contemporary Japanese Culture. North Clarendon, VT: Tuttle.

De Lange, F., 2011. Restoring Autonomy. Symmetry and Asymmetry in Care Relations. *Nederduitse Gereformeerde Teleogiese Tydskrif* 52, 61–68.

Douglas, M., 1990. Foreword. No Free Gifts. *In:* Mauss, M. ed. *The Gift. The Form and Reason for Exchange in Archaic Societies.* London: Routledge, vii–xviii.

Ehrnrooth, J., 1995. *Asentoja. Muistelmia nykyajasta.* Helsinki: WSOY.

Ehrnrooth, J., 2014. *Toivon tarkoitus.* Helsinki: Kirjapaja.

Engdahl, H., 2013. *Ja sen jälkeen savuke.* Helsinki: Siltala. (Original: Meteorer. Stockholm: Albet Bonniers Förlag, 1999.)

Fisher, B., and Tronto, J., 1990. Toward a Feminist Theory of Caring. *In:* Abel, F. and Nelson, M. eds. *Circles of Care.* Albany: State University of New York, 35–62.

Gérard-Veret, L. A., Kolm, S. C., Ythier, J., and Mercier, J. eds. 2000. *The Economics of Reciprocity, Giving and Altruism.* Basingstoke: Macmillan Press.

Gintis, H., 2000a. Beyond Homo Economicus: Evidence from Experimental Economics. *Ecological Economics* 35:311–322.

Gintis, H., 2000b. *Strong Reciprocity and Human Sociality.* Amherst: University of Massachusetts, Economics Department working Paper series 82.

Gouldner, A. W., 1960. The Norm of Reciprocity: A Preliminary Statement. *American Sociological Review* 2, 161–178.

Grenier, A., and Phillipson, C., 2013. Rethinking Agency in Late Life: Structural and Interpretive Approaches. *In:* Baars, J., Dohmer, J., Grenier, A., and Phillipson, C., eds. *Ageing, Meaning and Social Structure. Connecting Humanistic and Critical Gerontology.* Bristol: Policy Press.

Haapola, I., Vaara, E., and Karisto, A., 2013. Koettu hyvinvointi. *In:* Haapola, I., Karisto, A. and Fogelholm, M., eds. *Vanhuusikä muutoksessa. Ikihyvä Päijät-Häme-tutkimuksen tuloksia 2002–2012.* Päijät-Hämeen sosiaali- ja terveysyhtymän julkaisuja 72, 83–90.

24   *Antti Karisto*

Hirvilammi, T., 2015. Kestävän hyvinvoinnin jäljillä. Ekologisten kysymysten integroiminen hyvinvointitutkimukseen. Helsinki: Kela, Sosiaali- ja terveysturvan tutkimuksia 136.

Honneth, A., 2005. *The Struggle for Recognition. The Moral Grammar of Social Conflicts.* Cambridge: Polity Press.

Jaakkola, L., 2008. *"Mitäs sulle?" Kohtelias asiakaspalvelu ikääntyvien ja ikääntyneiden tulkinnoissa.* Soveltavan kielentutkimuksen lisensiaattityö. Jyväskylän yliopisto.

Jalava, J., and Kangas, R., 2013. Kommunikaatio, yhteiskunnan eriytyminen ja osasysteemien merkitys. *In:* Jalava, J., ed. *Yhteiskunnan järjestelmät. Niklas Luhmannin ajattelu.* Helsinki: Gaudeamus, 40–59.

Johansson, S., 1979. *Mot en teori för social rapportering.* Stockholm: Institutet för social forskning, Rapport Nr 2 från levnadsnivåprojekt.

Karisto, A., 2010. Yksi piano vai kymmenen lehmää? Kirjoituksia arjen ilmiöistä. Helsinki: Gaudeamus.

Knight, L. W., 2005. *Citizen: Jane Addams and the Struggle for Democracy.* Chicago: University of Chicago Press.

Kolm, S. C., 2000a. Introduction: The Economics of Reciprocity, Giving and Altruism. *In:* Gérard-Veret, L. A., Kolm, S. C., Ythier, J., and Mercier, J., eds. *The Economics of Reciprocity, Giving and Altruism.* Basingstoke: Macmillan Press, 1–46.

Kolm, S. C., 2000b. The Theory of Reciprocity. *In:* Gérard-Veret, L. A., Kolm, S. C., Ythier, J. and Mercier, J., eds. *The Economics of Reciprocity, Giving and Altruism.* Basingstoke: Macmillan Press, 115–141.

Kolm, S. C., 2008. *Reciprocity. An Economics of Social Relations.* Cambridge: Cambridge University Press.

Kortteinen, M., 1982. *Lähiö. Tutkimus elämäntapojen muutoksesta.* Helsinki: Otava.

Koskiaho, B., 2014. *Kumppanuuden sosiaalipolitiikkaa etsimässä.* Helsinki: Suomen Setlementtiliitto.

Kröger, T., Karisto, A., and Seppänen, M., 2007. Sosiaalityö vanhuuden edessä. *In:* Seppänen, M., Karisto, A., and Kröger, T., eds. *Vanhuus ja sosiaalityö. Sosiaalityö avuttomuuden ja toimijuuden välissä.* Jyväskylä: PS-Kustannus, 7–15.

Kujala, A., and Danielsbacka, M., 2015. *Hyvinvointivaltion loppu? Vallanpitäjät, kansa ja vastavuoroisuus.* Helsinki: Tammi.

Lasch, C., 1979. *The Culture of Narcissism. American Life in an Age of Diminishing Expectations.* New York: W.W. Norton.

Leitner, S., 2003. Varieties of Familialism. *European Societies* 5, 353–375.

Levinas, E., 1996. *Etiikka ja äärettömyys. Keskusteluja Philippe Nemon kanssa.* Helsinki: Gaudeamus. (Original: Ethique et infini. Dialogues d'Emmmanuel Levinas et Philippe Nemo, 1981.)

Liukko, J., 2013. *Solidaarisuuskone. Elämän vakuuttaminen ja vastuuajattelun muutos.* Helsinki: Gaudeamus.

MacIntyre, A., 1999. *Dependent Rational Animals. Why Human Beings Need the Virtues.* Chicago and La Salle, IL: Open Court.

Manatschal, A., 2015. Reciprocity as a Trigger of Social Cooperation in Contemporary Immigration Societies? *Acta Sociologica* 3, 233–248.

Martela, F., 2012. *Caring Connections – Compassionate Mutuality in the Organizational Life of a Nursing Home.* Aalto University Publication Series, Doctoral dissertations 144/2012.

Mauss, M., 1999. *Lahja*. Helsinki: Tutkijaliitto. (Original: Essai sur de lon. Presses Universitaires de France, 1950.)

Naukkarinen, O., 2011. Tahdikkuus esteettis-eettisenä toimintaperiaatteena. *Tiede & Edistys* 4, 315–330.

Nussbaum, M., 2001. *The Fragility of Goodness: Luck and Ethics in Greek Tragedy and Philosophy*. Cambridge: Cambridge University Press.

Palomäki, S. L., and Toikko, T., 2007. Tekemisen ja kohtaamisen ristiriita vanhustyössä. *In:* Seppänen, M., Karisto, A., and Kröger, T. eds. *Vanhuus ja sosiaalityö. Sosiaalityö avuttomuuden ja toimijuuden välissä*. Jyväskylä: PS-Kustannus, 271–288.

Pahl, R., 2000. *On Friendship*. Cambridge: Polity Press.

Pilcher, J., 1995. *Age and Generation in Modern Britain*. Oxford: Oxford University Press.

Pinker, S., 2011. *The Better Angels of Our Nature: Why Violence Has Declined*. New York: Viking.

Pirhonen, J., 2015. Tunnustaminen ja sen vastavuoroisuus vanhustyössä. Gerontologia 29(1), 25–34.

Polanyi, K., 2001. *The Great Transformation: The Political and Economic Origins of Our Time*. Boston, MA: Beacon Press.

Raittila, H., 2001. *Canal Grande*. Helsinki: WSOY.

Said, E., 2011. *Orientalismi*. Helsinki: Gaudeamus. (Original: Orientalism, London: Penguin, 1977.)

Sennett, R., 1999. *The Corrosion of Character. The Personal Consequences of Work in the New Capitalism*. New York: W.W. Norton.

Sennett, R., 2003. *Respect in a World of Inequality*. New York: W.W. Norton.

Simmel, G., 2005. *Suurkaupunki ja moderni elämä. Kirjoituksia vuosilta 1895–1917*. Helsinki: Gaudeamus. (Original: Die Grossstädte und Geistesleben. Jahrbuch der Gehestiftung IX, 1903.)

Sipilä, J., 2011. Hyvinvointivaltio sosiaalisena investointina: älä anna köyhälle kalaa vaan koulutus! *Yhteiskuntapolitiikka* 4, 359–372.

Sortheix, F., 2014. *Values and Wellbeing: An Analysis of Country and Group Influences*. University of Helsinki, Publications of the Department of Social Research 2014: 5.

Taylor, C., 1992. *Multiculturalism and "the Politics of Recognition"*. Princeton, NJ: Princeton University Press.

Thompson, S., 2013. *Reciprocity and Dependency in Old Age. Indian and UK Perspectives*. New York: Springer.

Titmuss, R., 1970. *The Gift Relationship: From Human Blood to Social Policy*. London: George Allen & Unwin.

Turner, B., 1989. Ageing, Status Politics and sociological Theory. *British Journal of Sociology* 40, 588–606.

Wolff, J., and De-Shalit, A., 2007. *Disadvantage*. Oxford: Oxford University Press.

2 Creating well-being through reciprocal relationships

Maritta Törrönen

Introduction

This chapter discusses reciprocity in connection with well-being and welfare and depicts how it can be theoretically understood with respect to social work and social policy practices, which together create a social care system in a society. It critically analyses the power relationships and promotes the view that equality between different partners creates well-being and welfare. Thus, reciprocal social work challenges the well-known power combination between the social worker or caregiver and the user of services, client or care recipient. Similarly, with respect to social policy, the welfare state and the institutions are understood to supplement the mutual support of individuals on the societal level, for instance, in the form of social security. There are regulations and norms that tell us about the responsibilities and the duties of citizens but also indicate what kinds of rights and privileges they have in a certain society (Gouldner 1960, p. 169).

Reciprocity becomes visible when different communities imply different reciprocities of mutual help among their members and between each member and the member's community. A family, especially, is usually seen as a primary source of reciprocal services and affection. Moreover, the political and public sector as well as the idea of a welfare state include various traditional indicators of reciprocity in various forms of help, e.g. health, pension and education (Kolm 2008, pp. 1–2):

> For instance, a free, peaceful and efficient society requires the mutual respect of persons and properties – the police and self-defence could not suffice and are costly – and people would or could not so respect others if they were not themselves respected. This permits, in particular, the working of markets and organisations, which also requires a minimum of trust, honesty, promise keeping, or fairness – and mutual help in organisations –, which can only be reciprocal.
>
> (Kolm 2008, p. 1)

Good social relationships are sustained by reciprocity, which is not supported by oppressive norms but instead is a balanced and fair set of free, helpful acts. These reinforce emotional bonds and their intensities. (Kolm 2008, p. 2).

If reciprocity is based on equality, it creates a feeling of companionship, friendship or solidarity and helps people behave well towards one another. This, in turn, affects collective well-being and is a prerequisite for a caring democracy that diminishes inequality and increases people's quality of life. In social services, this means meeting people with respect, supporting their empowerment and increasing their well-being. Reciprocity includes actions that support one's self-interest and also actions without an immediate benefit that are more universal, namely, actions that incorporate the idea of all human beings as brothers or sisters (see Niiniluoto 2015).

In the book *Reciprocity*, which discusses political philosophy, Lawrence C. Becker (1990, p. 4) states that the concept of reciprocity is so broad that it is difficult to come to a consensus regarding its definition. For some, reciprocity simply refers to less direct or exact returns 'in kind', but others may use it to refer to indirect or not in kind exchanges. There is no consensus on whether it is an obligation or an ideal, whether it demands retaliation or good for good, whether it is connected to the concept of justice, or whether it conflicts with benevolence (*ibid.*, p. 4). Because life can also be viewed as complicated and often contradictory – as Pierre Bourdieu (1990, p. 139) puts it, 'The complexity lies in the social reality' – the concepts of reciprocity contain many components too. Some also use 'reciprocity' when referring to its opposite, when one revenges or acts badly towards others, as non-reciprocity (for instance, see Pereira *et al.* 2005).

In this chapter, reciprocity is understood as a positive concept that can refer to direct or indirect exchange between individuals, communities and societies. I understand reciprocal acts, i.e. fairness, justice or good behaviour, as ideals. Moreover, the aims of welfare state, with respect to everyday life interactions, that reciprocity supports the well-being of both people and their communities. However, reciprocal acts might also sometimes entail a feeling resembling an obligation and thus include negative features that seem to limit the freedom to choose. This indicates my understanding of life and how it simultaneously contains happiness and sorrow as well as justice and injustice.

In recognition of the complex nature of reciprocity, in this chapter, I will draw on the social sciences and philosophy to develop my own conceptualisation of reciprocity, which includes my proposed dimensions, namely, *practical*, *symbolic* and *moral*. These aspects clarify the power relationships: How are the resources divided between people (practical dimension), who is accepted as part of the group or society (symbolic dimension) and who has real possibilities to choose (moral dimension)? In my earlier writings on reciprocity, I have noticed that most authors connect reciprocity to other concepts, e.g. the quality of an interaction, or use it interchangeably with non-reciprocity. In my view, the social-scientific definition of reciprocity, including both social work and social policy, in its most accurate form, addresses the well-being of humans and manages to simultaneously include all of the following elements: survival, togetherness and morality.

These ideas of reciprocity, which are based on the understanding that human beings are interdependent, serve as criticisms of the current global trends that demand complete self-sufficiency from people or similarly focus on their own economic prosperity (see Nussbaum 2011, pp. 10, 29, Sen 2009). Therefore, reciprocity is not only accepting that people are equal – it is also understanding that they have a voice that can be heard (Brooks 2012, p. 28). In other words, people are met in similar situations according to the ideas of universalism but also taken into consideration when they have special needs. In addition to exploring reciprocity, this chapter outlines the arguments against the idea that human beings always choose whatever will benefit themselves the most (see also Nussbaum 2011, pp. 10, 29, Sen 2009). It will indicate the complexity of human cooperation, which is a combination of selfishness or self-interest and integrity: the act of surpassing one's own interests and relying on reciprocity in the ongoing negotiations of everyday life.

The idea of reciprocity

Every society has norms of reciprocity. Examples include gift-giving rituals between lovers and friends, patterns of family life, the obligations of citizenship, and contracts. The details vary depending on time and place, but there is always some understanding of reciprocity and an intricate etiquette. Becker points out that reciprocity is often associated with utility or obligation: A benefit that has not been requested by the recipients obligates them to return the favour. It also appears that the greater the nature of the benevolent action, the stronger the sense of obligation is to repay it in kind. The obligation may be viewed as oppressive, a source of resentment or a source of delight, and these feelings can be either volatile or stable. This kind of alternation is a normal part of life and does not eliminate social injustice (Becker 1990, p. 73).

Positively understood, reciprocity contains the assumption that good acts accumulate reciprocally and that people can treat each other well. This is interlinked with the impression that human beings have universal characteristics all over the world. In the history of Western thought, such a suggestion is often defended with religious arguments (Niiniluoto 2015, pp. 277–279). Becker's concept of reciprocity has a religious slant, although it can also be understood as an ethical norm for human beings:

> ... that we should return good for good, in proportion to what we receive; that we should resist evil, but not do evil in return; that we should make reparation for the harm we do; and that we should be disposed to do those things as a matter of moral obligation.
>
> (Becker 1990, p. 4)

Becker's definition views reciprocity as containing elements of both what we can do and what we ought to do. His definition of reciprocity argues that, first, we owe a return for all the good we receive; it does not infer that we have to accept the good we have received. Second, although reciprocity should not be understood as obligatory, it may dispose the receiver towards reciprocation. Third, the sense of obligation may not be apparent at the moment of the reciprocal action, but the receiver may feel retrospectively that he or she has to return good with good. Reciprocity may be viewed as a debt that cannot be repaid and as a mortgage on the love of one's relatives and friends (Becker 1990, pp. 4–6).

Becker's definition is similar to the 'Golden Rule', which is espoused in many religions. For Christians, this is defined by the following words of Jesus: 'Do unto others as you would have them do unto you'. The Golden Rule is sometimes understood as reciprocal egoism: It combines service and the debt of gratitude in a similar way to a business negotiation (Niiniluoto 2015, pp. 277–278). It guides us to think not only of our own benefit but also of how we behave towards other people.

If reciprocity is a source of well-being or welfare, its opposite, non-reciprocity, can be deemed harmful and thus to decrease well-being and willingness to commit to solidary actions. It does not support the actions that create equality nor does it support participation. Reciprocity correlates with long and predictable relationships and trust, while non-reciprocity expresses distrust, which alienates people and decreases their willingness to help and support each other (see Harisalo and Miettinen 2010, pp. 13–15, 23, see also Kouvo 2010, p. 171).

On the individual level, non-reciprocity means that a person or a group of people value themselves over someone else. In other words, they protect their own interests and behave badly towards others, e.g. they bully, hate or act mean towards one another. Without trust, people's attitudes towards others are hostile, fearful, judgemental, contemptuous and isolationist. Non-acceptance, as a form of non-reciprocity or anti-reciprocity, excludes a person from the social community and the pleasures it may offer. This may create painful and stressful experiences, such as discrimination (see Lindenberg *et al.* 2010, McCormic 2009). Although, even if a group does have a a strong sense of solidarity, it can harm individual members or the whole society if a group or community is too closed; cases of sectarianism, racism and corruption serve as examples. (Allardt 1976, pp. 37–38, 42–46).

In addition, different societies at different times have identified the nature of human beings as egoistic, altruistic or capable of acting for others. A number of researchers (Lindenberg 2010, p. 27, Lindenberg *et al.* 2010, p. 9; see also Fetchenhauer and Dunning 2010, p. 61) understand solidary behaviour as containing altruism because people help others in times of need, which entails some form of sacrifice. If people have unselfish motives and reciprocity is not regulated, this can be called reciprocal altruism (Manatschal 2015, p. 235). However, if we continuously sacrifice ourselves or if we are only giving or receiving, our relationships are not reciprocal. Such relationships can abuse the goodwill or kindness of the giving members. Such non-reciprocal relationships do not conform to the norms of reciprocity.

On the societal level, non-reciprocity can violate human rights or the sovereignty of states, or it can weaken other societies. The struggle between reciprocity and non-reciprocity is often visible in a society and in social interactions – for example, when people and members of communities treat each other very badly but still remain together, leading to a long-standing enmity between the involved parties (see Nussman 2011, p. 52, Seligman and Csikszentmihalyi 2000). In addition, goodness or badness can also be divided into natural badness and moral badness. Accidents, pain and suffering in the world are parts of the natural order of nature and have a physical or biological basis, such as natural catastrophes or disease. In contrast, other unfortunate or unpleasant events result from humans' wrong choices, which hurt them or others (Niiniluoto 2015, pp. 141–142). Natural catastrophes, too, can be caused by human beings. This kind of division of reciprocity and non-reciprocity does not justify a multifaceted reality but instead helps us understand what supports our well-being and what does not.

The multidisciplinary concept of reciprocity

The concept of reciprocity applies to many different fields. It is widely used in economics, the social sciences (especially social anthropology), psychology and social psychology, psychiatry, biology, religious science and history. The concept itself is multidisciplinary and even interdisciplinary, which highlights the varied ways in which the concept is applied. Different disciplines examine reciprocity on different levels as the interdependency among individuals, communities or societies.

Social work and social policy are tools used to strengthen reciprocal relationships on both personal and societal levels, based on the principles of the welfare state, such as solidarity, equality and support for employment. Research into reciprocity in social work and social policy can be seen as a contribution to international social welfare research, which focusses on well-being and the communities that hold people together (see Becker 1990, Ostrom and Walker 2003). Well-being describes individual experiences, whereas welfare refers to the support offered for well-being regulated by the state and other public or private services and benefits. Well-being can be defined by the experiences of individuals and groups, whereas welfare indicates the quality of life that is possible in a specific society. Reciprocal actions between individuals, communities and societies interact with one another, and as a result, well-being and welfare are created.

Reciprocity, then, refers to the interpersonal social and power relations within communities and societies. The concept is, therefore, much broader than the 'interactions between people': It includes emotional and evaluative functions. Kayongo Kabunda (1987, p. 33) defines reciprocity as interdependency. Therefore, reciprocity can be seen as 'universal dependence on the judgment of others' (see Bourdieu 2000, p. 100) that impacts both parties emotionally, e.g. liking each other. Reciprocal acts are motivated by the feelings of solidarity and affinity between persons or different groups who are engaged in the acts and give meaning and collective intentions to them. These acts connect people emotionally.

In social policy, the welfare state and institutions supplement the mutual support of individuals in a society. Regulations and norms define the citizens' responsibilities and duties but also their rights and privileges in a society. Similarly, in social work, this means that people can feel that they can influence their own lives, be important and feel respected (see Ojanen 2014, p. 313). They are supported when they need or ask for help, and there are no expectations of direct exchange. At times, situations also occur in which professionals have to act in the best interests of their clients. Therefore, reciprocity in social work can be seen as in relational social work, in which the helping process and the development of well-being are co-constructions: The contributions of both the social worker or caregiver and also the client or the care recipient are essential. Ideally, both are valued, supported and helped, and both are empowered by this system (Raineri and Cabiati 2015, p. 1, Thompson 2016, p. 14).

This understanding of reciprocity as in relation to social work and social policy contributes to the research tradition of social capital, which looks at changes within communities and the way in which well-being is socially created (Bourdieu 1984, Coleman 1990, Putnam 2000, Putnam *et al.* 1994). Social capital refers to social commitments and to changes in the sense of solidarity and emotional connectedness. It echoes and enhances interpersonal, social and global relationships (Coleman 1990, p. 2, Putnam *et al.* 1994, p. 167).

Both of these traditions, reciprocity and social capital, are rooted in the idea that people are inclined and, in fact, need to live in organised groups that promote the well-being of their members (Tuomela and Mäkelä 2011, p. 88). Further aspects include helping the society to function, increasing the happiness of its members and improving their health (Kouvo 2010, p. 166, Putnam *et al.* 1994, p. 169, Putnam 2000, p. 19). For instance, Raimo Tuomela and Pekka Mäkelä (2011, p. 88) claim that being social is the basis of human existence and is generally accepted by all people (see also Lindenberg and Steg 2007, Lindenberg *et al.* 2010). This trend reflects a strong collective intentionality – a 'we' mode that is at the core of social interactions (Tuomela and Mäkelä 2011, p. 90) and is connected to the collective well-being of individuals. Correspondingly, the social structures that maintain order and power cannot usually function without an authorisation from their citizens, who can offer their opinion, for instance, by voting or protesting.

In economics, reciprocity is associated with trading, selling and buying, and the theoretical approach to it is often based on an economic or a game theory (see Tuomela and Mäkelä 2011, p. 89). In the game theory, players follow certain rules and try to determine the best moves (Becker 1990, p. 7). The game theory is based on rational choices and the probability of accountability; it highlights the disharmonious nature of reciprocity – the struggle between benevolence and calculations (Törrönen 2012, p. 185).

The usual goals of business negotiations include financial benefits and growth. As for economics, and even the social sciences, many people hold strong opinions that highlight 'against payment' and reimbursements of benefits (see Kildal 2001, p. 2). Such views support the idea of man as an egoist, thinking only of his own benefit (see, for instance, Bierhoff and Fetchenhauer 2010, p. 226, Fetchenhauer and Dunning 2010, p. 72, Homans 1974). Marii Paskov's work (2016, pp. 4–5) serves as an example; she sees solidary actions as attempts to gain appreciation and honour or to elevate one's social status. Marcel Mauss had a similar viewpoint at the beginning of the 20th century, when he developed the idea of a gift, which is based on the research conducted among certain tribes and on their exchanges of gifts. Based on his anthropological research, he claims that there are no disinterested gifts. Mauss (2002) argues that all presents and acts of honour are made for certain purposes: to gain more acceptance and honour in the givers' communities.

Although recent global trends seem to strongly support this kind of egoistic understanding of human beings and their actions, many everyday experiences as well as research (see, for instance, Bierhoff and Fetchenhauer 2010, p. 226) also support the idea that people help and support one another without any immediate benefits. Becker (1990, p. 10) views reciprocity as a moral argument that does not offer the degree of precision required in mathematics. Amartya Sen (2009, pp. 32, 189) also underlines the importance of considering one's self-interest but also how the lives of others could be affected by one's actions.

Reciprocity is closely associated with several concepts from social psychology, such as 'sociability, social networks, social support, trust, community and civic engagement, helping and solidarity' (Morrow 1999, p. 744). Social support, then, is connected to reciprocity and can be defined as mutual or shared interventions or actions that have emotional, evaluative and informative dimensions. People who support one another feel the reciprocal nature of their interactions and the ways they are evaluated; the information they gain helps them to relate to others. Reciprocal relationships, including social support, make people's existences in the world more confident.

Reciprocity is also similar to the multidisciplinary concept of solidarity used, for instance, in sociology when a society considers it important to help people in need, to support mutual wellness with acts of kindness, to trust others and to be fair (see Fetchenhauer and Dunning 2010, p. 61, Lindenberg *et al.* 2010, p. 3). Reciprocity demands a negotiable relationship with frequent mutual actions that improve the possibility of survival. Reciprocal acts may be ongoing, random or repeating, and their temporal dimension always has an impact on the partners' relationships. Acts of reciprocity when someone is in need or in crisis also contain temporal and solidary elements.

Martha Nussbaum (2011, pp. 10–11) postulates from the philosophical point of view that when children experience vulnerability in various situations, they concurrently develop vivid imaginations and learn about other people. Thinking and imagination enrich relationships. Through this process, children learn how to treat others as equals and understand the meanings of reciprocal actions; without this process, they would only use others for their own gains. Nussbaum claims that if the citizens of a democracy lack empathy, they are inevitably more likely to exclude and stigmatise outsiders. The political struggle for liberty and equality requires that empathy, love and respect triumph over fear, jealousy and self-centred hostility, as Mahatma Gandhi described in his ideals for building a democracy (Nussbaum 2011, pp. 10–11, 20, 45, 165).

Nussbaum's understanding of how humans grow in a democratic society incorporates psychological theories, especially the attachment theory (Bowlby 1997; see also Brazelton and Cramer 1991), wherein reciprocity is often linked to interpersonal relationships. Douglas Hazel (2007, p. 46) points out that in developmental psychology, the parent-child relationship can be described as a dance that has certain steps. Reciprocity is expressed in the rhythm of the dance and in the smiles that communicate acceptance and benevolence from parent to child and vice versa. This can also be seen as a game, with predictable rules and two participants whose actions respond to one another's behaviour (Hazel 2007, p. 48).

The dimensions of reciprocity

Here, power is understood in relation to human beings who control one another and thus create boundaries: how the resources are divided in the world and between people (practical dimension), who is accepted as part of 'us' (symbolic dimension) and who has a real possibility to choose (moral dimension). This is based on the understanding that there are no empty systems or institutions but, conversely, that there are people who lead the institutions and have the power to make decisions and people who follow their rules. However, we cannot exclude ourselves because there are also responsibilities and rights in the society, which include us too.

We need resources with which to satisfy our basic needs (see, for instance, Maslow 1954); we need other people to share our lives and make moral decisions that support our and our communities' well-being. These elements are here called 1) practical dimension, 2) symbolic dimension and 3) moral dimension, which are combined with resources, social bonds and moral actions. The dimensions create a multidimensional picture of our well-being. These dimensions overlap with one another, addressing the equality of human beings in the material, social and moral senses and describing

Table 2.1 Practical, symbolic and moral dimensions of reciprocity

Dimensions	Areas	Outcomes	Well-being
Practical	Resources	Survival and self-realisation	Material, physical and mental
Symbolic	Social bonding	Recognition, belonging and legitimisation	Social and emotional
Moral	Moral actions	Choices	Existential

the kinds of inequalities that individuals might encounter in everyday lives (Table 2.1).

First, without resources like food, shelter and finances, we could not survive, much less thrive or self-realise. Second, in our social relationships, we need to be recognised and feel that we belong and have the opportunities and entitlement to act in our societies (legitimisation). Third, nevertheless, people as moral actors and within certain limits can affect their own lives and, at the same time, the well-being of others. Taken together, these dimensions affect our well-being materially, physically, mentally, socially, emotionally and existentially. The extents to which we can influence our own lives and make choices affects how we experience our existences in the world. Together, these three dimensions of reciprocity have profound ontological significance for individuals and for the function of communities.

These dimensions resemble the division of needs described by Finnish sociologist Erik Allardt (1976): *having, loving* and *being,* which describe wealth, social security and individual existence as sources for well-being (see Niiniluoto 2015, p. 190). This chapter suggests the following difference: Reciprocity is not solely based on needs, resources or social bonds, but it also includes an understanding of a human being as a social and moral actor (see Niemelä 2010, pp. 19, 29). How individuals, communities and societies interact, and make commitments impacts their well-being and the welfare of their communities as a whole.

Good social relationships, both interpersonal and intergenerational, are very important for the well-being of humans. That is the reason for adding the symbolic dimension here (see also Törrönen 2015). If people take care of each other, treat each other well and are ready to commit to reciprocal acts, even love, these acts increase their well-being. I share Sanford C. Goldberg's opinion (2012, pp. vi–vii, 1) that we depend on one another very much. We find our own places and meanings in the world, based on our relationships with other people and on the human collectives that are close to us or that impact our lives. Our concepts of our own places and the meanings of our existences also depend on the understanding of how we are valued and recognised in these relationships and how our actions are accepted and the consequent effects they have.

Practical dimension

Historically, in social work and social policy, there has been an understanding that some problems are related to the uneven distribution or exchange of resources based on, e.g., social status, wealth, gender, ethnic origin or religion. This gives rise to the following question: Is the aim of sharing to reach equality or not? As Stephen Hawking (2016) puts it,

> Perhaps in a few hundred years, we will have established human colonies amid the stars, but right now we only have one planet, and we need to work together to protect it. To do that, we need to break down, not build up, barriers within and between nations. If we are to stand a chance of doing that, the world's leaders need to acknowledge that they have failed and are failing the many. With resources increasingly concentrated in the hands of a few, we are going to have to learn to share far more than at present.

The uneven distribution of power and wealth is understood to create inequality; people settle into hierarchical positions based on cultural, economic (Bourdieu 1984, [Bourdieu uses capital]) and health-related resources (Törrönen 2016, see also Törrönen 2014). These resources are affected by power relationships and structures. Such social structures include patriarchy, racism, capitalism and heterosexuality, which can be understood as primary structures. The secondary structures include family, community and bureaucracy, which include the media, the educational system and the authorities (Carniol 1992, p. 5). The resources of the practical dimension here are cultural, economic and health resources. Examples of economic resources include housing, work, subsistence and the standard of a home. Cultural resources include religion or ideology, education, family background and upbringing. Health-related resources include both physical and mental health. Inequality demonstrates the differences in power relations that are created by differences regarding the divisions of labour and knowledge but also by differences in cultural habits and social norms, which are considered valuable in certain places and at certain times.

Resources are used with respect to direct or indirect exchange, for instance, when taking care of others or offering food to others. If they are equally shared, they give individuals opportunities to satisfy their own needs and have the freedom to act. This is not self-evident, as Bourdieu puts it. He makes it clear that individuals cannot single-handedly determine the social positions they attain or their levels of freedom and equality in society; there is an ongoing struggle for resources. In addition to resources, there are some practical rules that shape human behaviour. These rules determine the following aspects: who in a certain culture has the opportunity to participate and what is prioritised; what is permissible, valued or procedurally correct; and, finally, how the rules are transformed or legitimised (Becker 1990, pp. 14–16).

Equality in a society depends on how the resources are shared, what kind of a social and healthcare system exists, and how this system takes care of people in need and during difficult times, e.g. regarding people who are unemployed or immigrants. An uneven distribution of resources usually lies behind inequality; however, there are also other disparities that affect well-being. The growth of inequality reflects collective attitudes towards the causes of difficulties and diminishes reciprocal actions.

The practical dimension describes how resources are shared in communities. It does not sufficiently clarify the concept of reciprocity in all of its dimensions (see Becker 1990, pp. 14–16, Sen 2009, pp. 233, 253). We need to also understand a human being as a social creature.

Symbolic dimension

The symbolic dimension addresses social and emotional well-being in making social bonds, which can be described as social resources. It simultaneously illustrates the opinion formed by the majority and the power relationships in a society. It describes how the members of the society are recognised and appreciated. Social bonds include intergenerational and other types of relationships. As Nussbaum (2011, p. 20) states, another human being should be met as a soul, not only as a useful tool or an obstacle to one's own plans. The symbolic dimension represents collective involvement and acceptance of others – the social bonding that creates a personal experience of social status in a certain community.

Here, I have modified the symbolic dimension to include recognition, belonging and legitimisation, which I define similarly to Bourdieu's definition of symbolic power (see Törrönen 2015). Bourdieu (1990, p. 138) defines symbolic power, first, as the credit or power granted to those who have sufficient recognition to be in a position to recognise others and, second, as the power to create things with words. Symbolic power contains elements of recognition and the justification for cooperative competition as a justification for existence, here called 'recognition', 'legitimisation' and 'belonging' (or participation).

The symbolic dimension describes how reciprocal actions, interaction and cooperation with others support our well-being. Therefore, an individual existence is a combination of circumstances outside the individual's control and aspects the individual can influence (Heidegger 2000, pp. 31, 41, 158–159, 289). This interprets people as active actors, not just passive respondents, and thus their motives influence their actions (Törrönen 2016, pp. 44–48). Motives include the possible outcomes of an action, based on one's values and priorities. Motives may be short term or hedonistic ('to feel better right now'), long term ('to improve one's resources') or normative ('to act appropriately') (Lindenberg 2010, p. 12), which helps explain why an individual's behaviour is sometimes difficult to predict, understand or grasp.

People do not only act with others in mind, they want to be valued in these relationships. Being valued creates an awareness to be collectively recognised. *Recognition* is connected to human dignity when one feels valued by certain people or communities. Metaphorically, this refers to a person's becoming visible 'in the eyes of others' (Pulkkinen 2002, p. 42). In Bourdieu's (2000) thinking, collective recognition is the fundamental existential goal of finding the meaning of life and the symbolic competition in lifestyles that maintain momentum in a society. The symbolic competition works to exclude or distinguish the social positions of people or communities in a power struggle (see Bourdieu 1990, pp. 123, 128–129, 2000, pp. 134–135). The symbolic dimension includes the emotional experiences and identities that make some people, geographical areas, ideologies or religions more familiar, closer and emotionally more touching for a person or persons (see Törrönen 1999, p. 23, Tuan 1987, p. 29). Sometimes, it is enough if there is at least one person who sees one's worth. These experiences and identities tend to create social hierarchies or polarisations between people and are created in reflexive interactions with others in long-lasting processes.

The relations are built up with sympathy and antipathy. Bourdieu (1990, p. 128; see also Sen 2009, pp. xvii, 39) writes that sympathy and antipathy, as means of distinction and emotional experience, set the foundation for all forms of cooperation, friendship, love affairs, marriages and associations. Like-minded people can more easily understand one another; this includes the acceptance of common rules, practices and institutions. These like-minded people are willing to meet expectations and share their experiences with others. This may take various forms: e.g. mutually shared opinions, controlling others, conciliation, negotiations, individual rights or respect (Azarian 2010, pp. 236–327). The social relations and mutual liking give rise to the sources of the symbolic competition that keep society in an endless motion (see Gabriel 2011, p. 3). Such a competition refers to the legitimacy of one's existence, namely, the individual right to feel justified in existing as one exists (Bourdieu 2000, p. 237).

Although fellow human beings value and like a person, he or she needs a feeling of *belonging*. This is a feeling of involvement and participation, of being connected to different social networks and other people through mutual obligations. It can also be a sense of emotional togetherness with a wider community based on e.g. suburb, nation, wealth, social class, disability, religion, sexual orientation, ethnic background, generation, gender (see also Nussbaum 2011, p. 24), society or even continent.

The interaction between members may strengthen the feeling of belonging together; it may also produce social ties, which makes life feel richer (Putnam 2000, p. 19). It is assumed that people return social support in proportion to their experiences of receiving it in their communities (see Newcomb 1990); however, people can also give more or less than they have received. This means that not everything can be calculated by money or volume; instead, belonging to some type of social capital can be very important for one's wealth, work satisfaction, health and ability to participate in a functioning democratic system (see Kouvo 2010, p. 166). Social capital supports the idea that well-functioning communities support the welfare of the whole society.

In addition to recognition and belonging, one's existence and obligations require a certain degree of collective acceptance and communal lawfulness. This can be called *legitimisation*, which provides individuals with the opportunities and the entitlement to act in a society, regulating the forms and intensity of cooperation among people and communities. If people have clear intentions and consequently fulfil their obligations in fair arrangements, others tend to trust and have confidence in them (Sen 2009, p. 80). This clarifies the power relationships (see Sennett 2003) in a society and in communities, in other words, who accepts and who is asking for acceptance.

The well-being of human beings is affected by the available resources in use and the natures of their social relationships but also by the kinds of possibilities they have to choose from and make decisions concerning their own lives. Moreover, we are moral actors, who simultaneously have certain rights and follow collective orders to participate in societies or in specific groups but also to consider how to meet responsibilities in societies or communities.

Moral dimension

There is no universal consensus on moral norms. Moral norms are learned in a reflexive process from childhood to adulthood, for instance, how the person respects another person's integrity or property. The norms also create tension between different actors because of (for example) religious or other ideological differences. The dominant moral obligations and codes, controlled by habits of thought, propensities to act and readiness to respond (Becker 1990, p. 37, see also Niiniluoto 2015, p. 178) in a society form the collective way of life. This way of life can be seen in the choices that individuals make as moral actors. This does not mean that they totally choose the way of life; it shows that human beings have the moral capacity to think and choose. This dimension separates people from animals; the practical and symbolic dimensions of reciprocity, or something similar, can also be observed in some animal communities (see, for instance, Honkalinna 2015).

People are disposed towards reciprocity in social practices (Becker 1990, p. 17). If a person acts against the moral norms of the community, the person might feel guilty afterwards or lose honour or trust in the eyes of the community (Niiniluoto 2015, p. 179). When combined with moral responsibilities, reciprocity motivates the people living in one particular area or people who are considered as a unit because of their common interests, social group, or nationality (see Cambridge Dictionary 2017). For instance, an employer usually pays a worker's salary, not only because they have an agreement but also because the employer sees that the employee deserves it. The act of the employer can be understood as a responsibility but also as a repayment to the employee. The norm of reciprocity requires that you do your part when others have completed theirs (Gouldner 1960, p. 175). However, Alvin W. Gouldner (1960, p. 170) does not consider the social practices to completely explain human behaviour, e.g. the interdependence connected to the division of labour; an individual sense of moral considerations and reciprocal actions also have an influence.

Becker (1990, p. 17) claims that morality is not a question of a choice: It is a way of life in which what we do is what we ought to do. He views morality as comprising not only purposeful actions but also states of being that conform to moral judgments. He draws on a virtue theory, also called a moral theory, to justify his views on reciprocity. The moral theory defines and justifies a proper way of life and the manners that moral agents should use. Becker favours the general concept of morality: '*moral judgments are judgments about what rational agents ought to do or be...*' (Becker 1990, p. 17). According to his moral theory, the general idea of morality, together with hedonic values, underpins personal welfare and efficiency. According to this theory, the moral argument will favour the better option due to the valuation of rules. As noted by Becker, '*better, on any given scale, is preferable to worse*' (Becker 1990, pp. 16, 37, 45, 73–74).

In an ethical sense, moral rules tell us how to behave and how to relate to other people and their communities and oblige us to behave in this way. Morality is created inside human communities, while laws have a history and were created by specific people. Several optional norms can exist simultaneously in the moral dimension (Niiniluoto 2015, p. 179), which can create tension between individuals. Ilkka Niiniluoto (2015, pp. 141–146) states that people are morally responsible for acting according to moral norms, which are reinforced by criminal laws that legally punish socially unacceptable acts. Moral norms are personal convictions and commitments; it is natural for people to seek their own benefits as long as they do not harm others. On the other hand, selfish, greedy acts that do not take other people into account are immoral. Consequently, a moral attitude cannot be limited to self-advantage because it should consider other people to be equal to oneself (*ibid.* pp. 141–146, 178–179).

Also, one's personality impacts one's moral acts. We have persistent tendencies in acting, reacting and responding. Consequently, there are also positive and negative reciprocators. Positive reciprocators are highly reactive to other people's behaviour and are additionally concerned with joint outcomes. Negative reciprocators are seen as more reactive to exchanges, which involves an ability to punish the other or 'get even' in an interpersonal exchange (Van der Zee and Perugini 2010, pp. 87–88).

Individual preferences do not always correspond to their judgments about what to do and who to be. If they did, conflicting attitudes, feelings and preferences would be automatically resolved. Unfortunately, this is not possible. Individuals have different opinions about the same aspects, and their reasons and emotions may vary. Because our lives are full of competing aims, values, ideals and demands, which lead to issues of prioritisation, and because one is not completely pure at the level of the heart, one competes for resources (Becker 1990, pp. 38–39; 42–44).

Sen has pointed out a very crucial element for being in the world: the importance of the freedom to choose. He does not, however, believe that everyone has the freedom to choose his or her own life (Sen 2009, pp. 18–19, see also Sartre 1957, p. 15):

> The freedoms and capabilities we enjoy can also be valuable to us, and it is ultimately for us to decide how to use the freedom we have.
>
> (Sen 2009, p. 19)

Sen's idea of freedom to choose is very important: The person has the freedom to choose if she has that opportunity in real life. How well we can make decisions concerning our own lives, how satisfied we may feel in following our own aspirations and goals, impacts our well-being. Consequently, if we feel that we have the right to exist as we are, for instance, if we feel that others appreciate our work or our actions for the common well-being of our families, we can feel existential well-being. Unfortunately, this brings constant inner and outer contradictions into our lives. We have to try to continuously find a balance between our own wishes and the obligations with which we are encircled.

Conclusion

We are strongly interdependent on each other in everyday life and also in the way that we understand our lives and the world around us (see Goldberg 2012, pp. vi–vii, 1). Reciprocal relationships support people with empowering feelings, such as love, empathy and resemblance, and give them strength to be loyal. Reciprocal relationships strengthen one's overall well-being and give meaning to one's life. However, experiences contain both reciprocal and non-reciprocal actions, and an individual may also act differently in different contexts.

When people experience togetherness, they are willing to display good gestures towards other members of their groups or societies. Reciprocity, therefore, can be understood as gestures or acts of goodwill that follow similar previous gestures or acts or alternatively are based on moral norms. Therefore, reciprocity can be seen as the prerequisite for life; it also maintains the obligations and ideals of communities and of social institutions and practices (Becker 1990, pp. 3–4). This kind of structure is also observable in a society: Do people feel togetherness in a society, and are they willing to support one another?

I understand that our everyday lives consist of both reciprocal and non-reciprocal experiences simultaneously. For instance, you may feel satisfied with some experiences in your own life but become worried about your friend's health or a crisis in your country. I agree with Gouldner (1960) that reciprocity is not only a kind of social interaction but the power that rules people and the world and regulates social behaviour. Globally, there seems to be a tendency to attribute experiences of good or bad to some persons or groups within a population and the accumulation of wealth or impoverishment to some others. This keeps us in the ongoing struggle to balance our well-being and find our own ways of life in the jungle of reciprocal and non-reciprocal relationships. I have defined reciprocity and non-reciprocity as follows:

Reciprocity is the fundamental basis for human life and is connected to subjectively interpreted well-being but also to welfare, which is offered by the society, with its services and social security systems. It is based on the understanding that human beings are interdependent, which gives them a feeling of quiet obligation to follow the social and moral norms of their communities. However, it contains acts of sympathy and goodwill, which follow each other, and which are based on trust and can surpass individuality and reach out to strangers. Reciprocal relationships make people feel equal and heard; they impact people's own life situations. Reciprocal experiences are strongly associated with feelings of love, empathy, gratitude and satisfaction.

The opposite of reciprocity is non-reciprocity, which describes people's inequalities in their communities, which create negativity and antipathy and can take the form of extreme contempt, abuse, violations of human rights or even exploitation. At its weakest, it is nonchalance or indifference. Here, people see others more as individual actors or even competitors who are accused when difficulties occur in their own lives, and, moreover, inequality in the world is taken for granted. Relationships are built up with the hierarchy and paternalism. Non-reciprocity creates situations in which people feel excluded, hurt, ignored and not heard. These kinds of situations generate anger, anxiety and helplessness.

The implications of reciprocal social work and social policy are that they clarify the importance of people's social relationships and commitments and can also examine their senses of solidarity and emotional connectedness (see Coleman 1990, p. 2, Putnam *et al.* 1994, p. 167). It may help to transform individualistic services into community empowerment that gives value, for instance, to peers and intergenerational relationships. Community work can mean reorganising services and their delivery but can also mean voluntary help and support without always having to use money, e.g., exchanges of services, support, help or company. This means that one's own knowledge and experiences are taken more into account when developing new health and social services.

At the same time, there is a strong need to strengthen an equal income distribution and fair distribution of other resources and services, which are ways of attaining societal reciprocity and maintaining status quo in societies; these objectives also support individual well-being. People who are in difficult life situations especially need the support of the welfare state because they might have less possibilities for reciprocal acts. Consequently, society functions better when respect and appreciation are commonly expressed.

On the societal level, democracy can be considered as a prerequisite for the welfare of human communities. If a society follows the rules of democracy and supports reciprocal acts, it increases equality among its citizens. The members of the society also have decent possibilities to care for each other, not only practically but also emotionally. Sen (2009, p. xiii) eloquently expresses the idea of a just society that creates good opportunities for reciprocity and thus promotes individual well-being: 'Democracy has to be judged not just by the institutions that formally exist but by the extent to which different voices from diverse sections of the people can actually be heard.'

References

Allardt, E., 1976. *Hyvinvoinnin ulottuvuuksia* [The Dimensions of Well-being]. Helsinki: WSOY.

Azarian, R., 2010. Social Ties: Elements of a Substantive Conceptualization. Acta Sociologica – Journal of the Nordic Sociological Association, 53 (4), 323–338.

Becker, L. C., 1990. *Reciprocity*. Chicago: University of Chicago Press.

Bierhoff, H. W. and Fetchenhauer, D., 2010. How to Explain Prosocial and Solidary Behavior: A Comparison of Framing Theory with Related Meta-Theoretical Paradigms. *In:* D. Fetchenhauer, A. Flache, A. P. Buunk and S. Lindenberg, eds. *Solidarity and Prosocial Behavior. An Integration of Sociological and Psychological Perspectives*. New York: Springer Science + Business Media, 225–242.

Bourdieu, P., 1984/1979. *Distinction. A Social Critique of the Judgement of Taste.* Cambridge: Harvard University Press.

Bourdieu, P., 1990. *In Other Words.* Stanford: Stanford University Press.

Bourdieu, P., 2000. *Pascalian Meditations.* Stanford: Stanford University Press.

Bowlby, J., 1997. *Attachment and Loss.* London: Pimlico.

Brazelton, T. B. and Cramer B. C., 1991. *The Earliest Relationship: Parents, Infants and the Drama of Early Attachment.* London: Karnac Books. Available from: https://helka.linneanet.fi/cgi-bin/Pwebrecon.cgi?BBID=2549117 [Accessed 14 Nov 2014].

Brooks, T., 2012. Reciprocity as Mutual Recognition. *The Good Society,* 14 (1), 21–26.

Cambridge Dictionary. Community. Available from: http://dictionary.cambridge.org [Accessed 10 Oct 2017].

Carniol, B., 1992. Structural Social Work. Maurice Moreau's Challenge to Social Work Practice. *Journal of Progressive Human Services* 3 (1), 1–20.

Coleman, J. S., 1990. *Foundations of Social Theory.* Massachusetts: The Belknap Press of Harvard University Press.

Fetchenhauer, D. and Dunning, D., 2010. Perceptions of Prosociality and Solidarity in Self and Others. *In:* D. Fechenhauer, A. Flache, A. P. Buunk and S. Lindenberg, eds. *Solidarity and Prosocial Behavior: An Integration of Sociological and*

Psychological Perspectives. Critical Issues in Social Justice. New York: Springer, 61–74.

Gabriel, P., 2011. The Social as Heaven and Hell. Pierre Bourdieu's Philosophical Anthropology. *Journal for the Theory of Social Behaviour*, 42 (1), 1–24. Available from: http://onlinelibrary.wiley.com/doi/10.1111/j.1468-5914.2011.00477.x/pdf [Accessed 14 Feb 2013].

Goldberg, S. C., 2012. *Relying on Others. An Essay in Epistemology.* Oxford: Oxford University Press.

Gouldner, A. W., 1960. The Norm of Reciprocity: A Preliminary Statement. *American Sociological Review*, 25 (2), 161–178.

Harisalo, R. and Miettinen, E., 2010. *Luottamus. Pääomien pääoma* [Trust – The Capital of the Capital]. Tampere: Tampere University Press.

Hawking, S., 2016. This is the Most Dangerous Time for Our Planet. Politics Opinion. *Guardian*. Available from: www.guardian.com [Accessed 6 Dec 2016].

Hazel, D., 2007. *Containment and Reciprocity: Integrating Psychoanalytic Theory and Child Development Research for Work with Children.* London: Routledge.

Heidegger, M., 2000. *Oleminen ja aika.* Tampere: Vastapaino.

Homans, G. C., 1974. *Social Behavior: Its Elementary Forms.* New York: Harcourt Brace Jovanovich.

Honkalinna, M. 2015. *Korppimatka.* Helsinki: Maahenki.

Kabunda, K., 1987. *Reciprocity and Interdependence. The Rise of the Kololo Empire in Southern Africa in the 19th Century.* Akademisk Avhandling av filosofie doktorsexamen vid Samhällsvetenskapliga fakulteten vid universitet i Lund. Lund: Studentlitteratur.

Kildal, N., 2001. *Welfare Policy and the Principle of Reciprocity.* Presentation at the Conference of International Sociological Association, Annual Conference, RC 19: Old and New Social Inequalities: What Challenges for Welfare States? Oviedo 6–9 September 2001, 16 pages.

Kolm, S. C., 2008. *Reciprocity. An Economics of Social Relations.* Cambridge: Cambridge University Press.

Kouvo, A., 2010. Luokat ja sosiaalinen pääoma. *In:* Erola, ed. *Luokaton Suomi. Yhteiskuntaluokat 2000-luvun Suomessa.* Helsinki: Gaudeamus, 166–181.

Lindenberg, S., 2010. Prosocial Behavior, Solidarity and Framing Processes. *In:* D. Fechenhauer, A. Flache, A. P. Buunk and S. Lindenberg, eds. *Solidarity and Prosocial Behavior: An Integration of Sociological and Psychological Perspectives. Critical Issues in Social Justice.* New York: Springer, 23–44.

Lindenberg, S., Fetchenhauer, D., Flache A., Buunk, A. P., 2010. Solidarity and Prosocial Behaviour: A Framing Approach. *In:* D. Fechenhauer, A. Flache, A. P. Buunk and S. Lindenberg, eds. *Solidarity and Prosocial Behavior: An Integration of Sociological and Psychological Perspectives. Critical Issues in Social Justice.* New York: Springer, 3–19.

Lindenberg, S. and Steg, L., 2007. Normative, Gain and Hedonic Goal Frames Guiding Environmental Behaviour. *Journal of Social Issues*, 63 (1), 117–137.

Manatschal, A., 2015. Reciprocity as a Trigger of Social Cooperation in Contemporary Immigration Societies? *Acta Sociologica*, 58 (3), 233–248.

Maslow, A. H., 1954. *Motivation and Personality.* New York: Harper and Brothers.

Mauss, M., 2002. *Lahja.* Helsinki: Tutkijaliitto.

McCormic, H., 2009. Intergenerational Justice and the Non-Reciprocity Problem. *Political Studies*, 57 (2), 451–458.

Morrow, V., 1999. Conceptualising Social Capital in Relation to the Well-Being of Children and Young People: A Critical Review. *The Sociological Review*, 47, 744–765.

Newcomb, M., 1990. Social Support by Many Other Names: Towards a Unified Conceptualization. *Journal of Social and Personal Relationships*, 7, 479–494.

Niemelä, P., 2010. Hyvinvointipolitiikan teoria. *In:* P. Niemelä, ed. *Hyvinvointipolitiikka*. Helsinki: WSOYpro, 16–37.

Niiniluoto, I., 2015. *Hyvän elämän filosofiaa*. Helsinki: Suomalaisen Kirjallisuuden Seura.

Nussbaum, M. C., 2011. *Talouskasvua tärkeämpää*. Miksi demokratia tarvitsee humanistista sivistystä. Helsinki: Gaudeamus. [Translation Timo Soukola].

Ojanen, M., 2014/2007. *Positiivinen psykologia*. Helsinki: Edita.

Ostrom, E. and Walker, J., eds., 2003. *Trust and Reciprocity: Interdisciplinary Lessons from Experiment Research*. A Volume in the Russell Sage Foundation Series on Trust. New York: Russell Sage Foundation.

Paskov, M., 2016. Is Solidarity less Important and less Functional in Egalitarian Contexts? *Acta Sociologica*, 59 (1), 3–18.

Pereira, P. T., Silva, N. and Silva, J. A., 2005. Positive and Negative Reciprocity in the Labor Market. *Journal of Economic Behavior & Organization*, 59, 406–422.

Pulkkinen, L., 2002. *Mukavaa yhdessä. Sosiaalinen alkupääoma ja lapsen sosiaalinen kehitys*. Jyväskylä: PS-Kustannus.

Putnam, R. D., *et al.*, 1994. *Making Democracy Work: Civic Traditions in Modern Italy*. New Jersey: Princeton University Press.

Putnam, R. D., 2000. *Bowling Alone: The Collapse and Revival of American Community*. New York: Simon and Schuster.

Sartre, J. P., 1957. *Existentialism and Human Emotions*. Canada: Kensington Publishing Corp, 9–53. Available from: http://www.philosophymagazine.com/others/MO_Sartre_ExistentialismG.htm [Accessed 27 March 2015].

Seligman, M. and Csikszentmihalyi, M., 2000. *Positive Psychology: An Introduction*. The Introduction to the Millennial Issue of the *American Psychologist*, 1–22. Available from: http://www.google.com/search?q=seligman+positive+psychology+an+introduction&rls=com.microsoft:fi&ie=UTF-8&oe=UTF-8&startIndex=&startPage=1&rlz=1I7ADFA_enFI440 [Accessed 22 March 2013].

Sen, A., 2009. *The Idea of Justice*. London: Penguin Books.

Sennett, R., 2003. *Respect in a World of Inequality*. New York: W.W. Norton & Company.

Thompson, S., 2016. Promoting Reciprocity in Old Age: A Social Work Challenge. *Social Work in Action*, 341–355. http://dx.doi.org/10.1080/09503153.2015.1135892. [Accessed 15 May 2016].

Tuan, Y. F., 1987. *Space and Place: The Perspective of Experience*. Minnesota: University of Minnesota Press.

Tuomela, R. and Mäkelä P., 2011. Sosiaalinen toiminta. *In:* T. Kotiranta, P. Niemi and R. Haaki, eds. *Sosiaalisen toiminnan perusta*. Helsinki: Gaudeamus, 87–112.

Törrönen, M., 1999. *Lasten arki laitoksessa*. Helsinki: Helsinki University Press.

Törrönen, M., 2012. Sosiaalityö ja arkinen hyvinvointi – vastavuoroisuuden dialektiikka [Social Work and Well-being – the Dialectics of Reciprocity]. *Janus*, 2 (20), 182–191.

Törrönen, M., 2014. *Everyday Happiness: The Everyday Well-Being of Families with Children*. Publications of the Department of Social Research 2014: 3. Helsinki: University of Helsinki.

Törrönen, M., 2015. Toward a Theoretical Framework for Social Work – Reciprocity: The Symbolic Justification for Existence. *Journal of Social Work and Ethics*, 12 (2), 77–88. Available from: www.jswve.org [Accessed 30 Oct 2015].

Törrönen, M., 2016. Vastavuoroisuuden yhteisöllinen luonne. *In:* M. Törrönen, K. Hänninen, P. Jouttimäki, T. Lehto-Lundén, P. Salovaara and M. Veistilä, eds. *Vastavuoroinen sosiaalityö.* Helsinki: Gaudeamus, 39–56.

Van der Zee, K. and Perugini, M., 2010. Personality and Solidary Behavior. *In:* D. Fechenhauer, A. Flache, A. P. Buunk and S. Lindenberg, eds. *Solidarity and Prosocial Behavior: An Integration of Sociological and Psychological Perspectives. Critical Issues in Social Justice.* New York: Springer, 77–92.

3 Reciprocity and normativity in social work

A complex relationship based on the Capability Approach

Bernhard Babic

Introduction

This chapter will focus on the interdependency between the concrete meaning of reciprocity for social work and the normative implications that inevitably come along with a certain understanding of social work. It will be explained why the first cannot be understood adequately without carefully reflecting on the latter.

Therefore, I will start with a few basic remarks on reciprocity. Then, in a second step, certain normative challenges of social work will be addressed. For a more specific and differentiated discussion of the related aspects, I will refer to the Capability Approach as a possible normative framework for social work and show some consequences of its application. Finally, I will present the conclusions that I derived from this example, concerning the relation between reciprocity and normativity.

Some brief remarks on reciprocity

Reciprocity is – as we have seen in the previous chapters – a very challenging and multifaceted subject. It can be understood as a synthesis of practical, symbolic and moral dimensions (see Törrönen, in this volume), with a significant influence on well-being (see Karisto, in this volume). Already, this illustrates to some extent its undeniable importance. Statements like 'Man becomes human in reciprocity' (Becker 1956, p. 94) or 'reciprocity (...) is the vital principle of society' (Hobhouse 1951, p. 12) emphasise its essential meaning for individuals and societies even more.

But beyond the fact that no one really seems to question the relevance of reciprocity, it is still unclear how to define it precisely (Gouldner 1960, p. 161, Perugini *et al.* 2003, p. 251). This certainly has something to do with the fact that many different disciplines (including sociology, sociobiology, sociopsychology, economics, anthropology and political science) refer to this term from their specific perspectives. It is hardly imaginable that one single definition could satisfy them all. So, in this chapter, I will not even try to come up with a solution for this issue. However, I will highlight some basic aspects of reciprocity, which seem to be relevant in the context of social work.

One of these aspects is, according to Alvin W. Gouldner, the necessity to at least distinguish between '(1) reciprocity as a pattern of mutually contingent exchange of gratifications, (2) the existential or folk belief in reciprocity, and (3) the generalized moral norm of reciprocity' (1960, p. 161).

Concerning reciprocity as a pattern of exchange of gratifications, Christian Stegbauer (2011, p. 28ff) differentiates four forms of reciprocity:

- Direct reciprocity, in this context, usually describes a direct exchange relation between two individuals. The receiving person directly rewards his giving counterpart, not necessarily immediately but ideally with something that both parties regard as equivalent or appropriate.
- Generalised reciprocity characterises an exchange in which the rewarded person is not the one who initiated the exchange, as is the case, e.g., when someone is asked to pay a received favour forward or when the giving person is seen as the representative of a group, which can have the consequence that another member of this group or the group as a whole benefits (or suffers) from the receiver's reciprocal behaviour.
- Reciprocity of positions refers to the fact that certain positions in society simply need a counterpart that justifies their existence, as in the case of physicians and their patients or in the analogy of social workers and their clients. These examples show that this kind of reciprocity can additionally often be characterised as asymmetrical because different positions within society can cause significant differences concerning the distribution of power within a certain situation. Therefore, it can happen that the receiving person is basically unable to return (directly) something equivalent. However, this is not necessarily the case when talking about this kind of reciprocity.
- Reciprocity of perspectives relates to people's abilities to imagine how somebody else thinks or feels about something. This is relevant, last but not least, for an appropriate assessment of someone's expectations within a reciprocal process.

The belief in reciprocity can be seen as a precondition in this context as it is not likely that people will reciprocate if they are not convinced that this is a reasonable behaviour that can be expected from others too.

Seen as a moral norm, reciprocity can be basically understood as the duty of returning a kindness (equivalently). Negatively formulated, it also to some extent justifies the revenge for unkind behaviour.

Although, of course, these basic reflections are not comprehensive or sufficient for defining reciprocity, it becomes obvious that reciprocity is indeed – as stated in the beginning – something very essential. According to Stegbauer (2011, p. 134ff), looking at reciprocity means nothing less than looking at some of the most important foundations of any social issue, including the society, because individuals and institutions are never the only constitutive elements. The relations between them are at least as important in this context, and they cannot be assessed appropriately without taking a closer look at the kind of reciprocity that is distinguishing them, as we can learn from network research (e.g. Stegbauer and Häußling 2010). As a consequence, this means that the kind of reciprocity that characterises relations in social work is also essential for an appropriate understanding and assessment of what is going on in this professional field.

Normative challenges

However, social work always encounters some normative challenges too. The fact that neither social work nor society confine themselves to securing their citizens' mere subsistence is one of the reasons for this. At least in wealthy economies, both are usually aimed at a higher standard of living. Because there is a growing discontent with the gross domestic product (GDP) as a measure in this context (see Stiglitz *et al.* 2008), more and more efforts can be observed to replace it by measuring people's well-being (e.g. OECD 2015). But concerning the concept of well-being, we seem to face comparable difficulties as those we faced already with the concept of reciprocity. Although its relevance is unquestionable, so far, there is also no generally accepted definition of it (see Karisto in this volume). At first glance, even the reasons for this lack of agreement seem to be quite similar. Well-being is, of course, an issue in many different disciplines (see Babic *et al.* 2017), and they all tend to define it according to their own perspectives and priorities. But, in contrast to reciprocity, there is at least one additional aspect, which seems to be less important when talking about reciprocity. While reciprocity (even as a norm) can be described more or less neutrally, e.g., as an observable behaviour that is taking place (or not) without being called good or bad, any concept of well-being includes inevitably explicit normative aspects. The term itself tells us that in the case of well-being, it's simply not enough to describe a certain way of being without any far-reaching expectations. It definitely has to be a label for a good way of being, which automatically raises the question 'what is good' or at least 'what is good enough'?

At this point, amongst others, David Hume's law reminds us that it is not appropriate to derive an 'ought' directly from an 'is' (see Russel 2010). Following this argument, it is more or less impossible for (empirical) science to answer the question above. And even if we do not agree with Hume's position and feel free to define an 'ought' scientifically, we cannot ignore the fact that scientists do not usually have the authorisation to determine what should be within pluralistic and democratic societies. For good reason, such decisions are a privilege of democratically legitimated parliamentarians.

This restriction, of course, applies to social workers too. To avoid being directed by others in this context, they are, as in any other profession, well advised to make suggestions concerning their professional normative orientations. But regardless of their explicit mandates to contribute to the improvement of their clients' lives and the normative implications of such activities (see Otto and Ziegler 2012), as professionals, social workers do not have the competence to decide on the normative orientations of their profession completely on their own as they (or their employers) usually act on behalf of the society. Therefore, the society – or at least its representatives – are finally responsible for defining the normative framework for social workers. And beyond this formal argument, in many instances, the profession is obviously far from being able to respond clearly or at least with one voice about how much and which normativity is necessary in social work (see Scherr 2012).

The Capability Approach

However, the Capability Approach (CA) has recently gained a lot of attention, especially within German-speaking discussions concerning the normative orientation of social work. This happened last but not least because it was already successfully implemented in various political fields and is basically compatible with social work (see Leßmann *et al.* 2014). Some supporters of the concept believe that it even has the potential to become the leading normative framework of the profession (see Otto and Ziegler 2006). But besides the fact that such assumptions can be questioned in general (see Babic 2011), one also has to be aware that the mentioned discussions are not always based on a sufficiently differentiated understanding of the approach (Babic and Leßmann 2016). Therefore, it might be helpful to introduce it briefly.

Following Bernhard Babic *et al.* (2010, p. 409f), the approach was originally formulated by the economist, philosopher and Nobel laureate Amartya Sen. It was explicitly meant as an alternative to neoliberal and utilitarian policy prescriptions in the field of human development. Accordingly, Sen suggests that we ask if and to what extent a certain development or intervention enables people to lead the kinds of lives they would really like to lead instead of basing assessments in this context primarily on such measures as the GDP, the growth of individual incomes, the availability of commodities or happiness (see Sen 2001). In other words, the CA puts a focus rather on what people are effectively able to do and be, that is, on their capabilities instead of what they have. This does not mean that income, happiness or commodities are not important. But from Sen's perspective, material resources, like income and commodities, are just means to an end, while happiness might be the consequence of a realised end. Therefore, it would be simply inadequate to refer only or primarily to one of these variables as an indicator for people's well-being within a policy or its evaluation.

In the end, this defines well-being as the opportunity to live life according to one's values. Additionally, it provides the degree of individual freedom to do so as a yardstick in this context. Agency, access to (material, social and environmental) resources, personal traits, abilities and knowledge to convert these resources into valuable beings and doings become necessary preconditions of well-being from this perspective. Sabina Alkire (2005, p. 1) illustrates this with the following example:

> if a program aims to maximize individual income, it may force indigenous people, subsistence farmers, or stay-at-home mothers to take paying jobs because otherwise they appear to have no income. The capability approach argues that focusing on freedom is a more accurate way to build what people really value. Focusing on freedom introduces fewer distortions.

This understanding, on the one hand, makes the assessment of well-being a task with a strong focus on the individual and his or her abilities and values. On the other hand, it is an emphasis on the individual's embeddedness in a society that is requested to offer him or her adequate options for achieving well-being. Both aspects can differ a lot and lead to very specific points of departures concerning the quest for well-being. As a consequence, Sen does not offer any kind of predefined list of generally relevant functionings[1] or capability sets.[2] These have to be defined specifically in each single case, and those who will be affected by a certain policy (or intervention) in the first place have to be involved in defining the relevant dimensions of well-being. The latter, of course, has to take place in a democratic process based on public reasoning (see Schokkaert 2008, p. 16ff).

In contrast to Sen, Martha Nussbaum, who claims that her version of the CA is a further development of Sen's original approach, offers a concrete list of ten central capabilities (see Nussbaum 2000, 2006).

Box 3.1 List of central functional capabilities (according to Nussbaum 2000, p. 78ff)

1 *Life*: being able to live to the end of a human life of normal length. Not dying prematurely or before one's life is so reduced as to be not worth living.
2 *Bodily health*: being able to have good health, including reproductive health; to be adequately nourished; to have adequate shelter.
3 *Bodily integrity:* being able to move freely from place to place; to be secure against violent assault, including sexual assault and domestic violence; to have opportunities for sexual satisfaction and for choice in matters of reproduction.
4 *Senses, imagination and thought:* being able to use the senses to imagine, think and reason – and to do these things in a truly human way, a way informed and cultivated by an adequate education, including, but by no means limited to, literacy and basic mathematical and scientific training. Being able to use imagination and

thought in connection with experiencing and producing works and events of one's own choice, which are religious, literary, musical and so forth. Being able to use one's mind in ways protected by guarantees of freedom of expression, with respect to both political and artistic speech and freedom of religious exercise. Being able to have pleasurable experiences and to avoid non-necessary pain.

5   *Emotions:* being able to have attachments to things and people outside ourselves; to love those who love and care for us, to grieve at their absences; in general, to love, to grieve and to experience longing, gratitude and justified anger. Not having one's emotional development blighted by fear and anxiety. (...)

6   *Practical reason:* being able to form a conception of good and to engage in critical reflection about the planning of one's life. (...)

7   *Affiliation:*

   A   Being able to live with and towards others; to recognise and show concern for other human beings; to engage in various forms of social interaction; to be able to imagine the situation of another and have compassion for that situation; to have the capability for both justice and friendship. (...)

   B   Having the social bases of self-respect and non-humiliation. Being able to be treated as a dignified being whose worth is equal to that of others. This entails protection against discrimination on the basis of race, sex, religion, caste, ethnicity or national origin.

8   *Other species:* being able to live with concern for and in relation to animals, plants and the world of nature.

9   *Play:* being able to laugh, to play and to enjoy recreational activities.

10   *Control over one's environment:*

   A   Political. Being able to participate effectively in political choices that govern one's life. Having the right of political participation, protections of free speech and association.

   B   Material. Being able to hold property (both land and movable goods). Having the right to seek employment on an equal basis with others. Having the freedom from unwarranted search and seizure.

To reach a sufficient level of well-being, it is necessary that all of these be realised to some extent, without any trade-offs between them. Although Nussbaum she admitted that her list is not comprehensive and can be changed, many criticised her for being quite paternalistic by universally determining capabilities for other cultures and societies (see Clark 2005, p. 7).

Additionally, at least in empirical sciences and related fields, the added value of Nussbaum's list can be questioned anyway as it usually needs further specification for an appropriate application (see Schokkaert 2008, p. 16f). Nevertheless, such lists are certainly useful for initiating debates on relevant dimensions of well-being.

However, the indicated differences between Sen's and Nussbaum's CA can be primarily explained by the different intentions they are following. Sen's version of the CA is mainly driven by his aim to improve the base for (international) comparisons of economies and the well-being they provide, while Nussbaum is primarily concerned with universally securing the suggested central capabilities (see above). Without going any further into details concerning the resulting disparities, I just want to highlight the different meaning of reciprocity that results from these two conceptions of the CA.

From Sen's perspective, reciprocity, primarily understood as a fundamental aspect that characterises our relations, can be regarded as an essential part of the individual's social resources as well as a conversion factor that allows or at least supports the realisation of well-being by achieving valued beings and doings. From Nussbaum's perspective, the issue is not that obvious as she is referring primarily to the state or to society as an entity that has to guarantee her universalistic central capabilities to all its citizens. One could argue that the notion of reciprocity is, to some extent, included by the fact that citizens and their reciprocal relations in return are forming the state and its institutions.

Potential consequences for social work and reciprocity

However, if one accepts the CA as a normative framework for social work, this also includes the approval that assessments of social work programmes or interventions have to be based primarily on the extent to which they really support people in living a 'good life'.

Operationalising the CA, according to Sen, could mean that social work has to first identify what a good life looks like from clients' points of view, with a high sensitivity to their specific values (e.g. Babic *et al.* 2010). It would be inevitable to involve clients actively in this process. As a consequence of such a participatory approach, social work cannot operate with precisely predefined goals. Taking further into account that realising a good life requires, on the one hand, that there be appropriate opportunities/freedoms to do so, which are last but not least something society has to provide (e.g. by according laws or institutions), and, on the other hand, the corresponding ability and willingness of an individual, social workers will have to pay attention to both aspects equally. Following this understanding and its normative implications, social work will be based on 'tailor made' flexible concepts and strategies (e.g. community-based approaches) rather than on highly standardised and institutionalised routines (e.g. evidence-based practices). Social work's task would be to support clients in developing their individual abilities to achieve valuable beings and doings according to their understandings of a good life as well as to work actively for the improvement of adequate opportunities for clients to do so within a society. From this point of view, an understanding of social work that refers to Sen's CA as a normative framework reveals a lot of commonalities with other up-to-date theories and concepts of the discipline and its practices. Although this does not answer all questions concerning an adequate operationalisation of the CA, one is able to get some first impressions of the possible outcomes of such efforts.

However, following Nussbaum's CA does not necessarily lead to similar evident results. Because of her lists of central capabilities, there seems to be a much bigger risk of ending up with a quite paternalistic concept of social work. For the sake of fairness, it is necessary to add that Nussbaum herself says that her list needs at least a specification when applied to a certain context and that, basically, it can be modified (even if she does not mention explicitly how). Nevertheless, controlling if and to what extent an individual reaches a sufficient level within each of the dimensions of a good life she predefined (no matter if the clients agree with her in this context or not) could be understood as a central task of the profession. Additionally, not reaching this level could be interpreted as a failure or an intolerable lack of willingness on the part of the individual. In this way, the list of central capabilities could even be (ab)used to limit the individual's freedom to pursue the realisation of his or her own understanding of a good and flourishing life by forcing him or her to develop primarily in Nussbaum's predefined areas. In fact, some authors reduce the CA because of the bigger paternalistic risks within Nussbaum's approach in general, which they view as a highly questionable attempt to instruct people in detail on how they should live (see Bossong 2011).

Of course, it can be questioned whether such a paternalistic interpretation of Nussbaum's intentions is appropriate. But here is unfortunately not the place to discuss this issue any further. The more important question in this context is about the relationship between normativity and reciprocity. And in this context, the simple differentiation between Sen and a paternalistic interpretation of Nussbaum already shows that looking at reciprocity alone does not necessarily provide significant information. Often, one will get a much better picture of what is really going on in social work when the normative orientation is taken into account too.

Concerning, for example, Stegbauer's four forms of reciprocity as a pattern of exchange of gratifications, it seems to be obvious that generalised reciprocity and reciprocity of positions are of high importance for social work. Clients do not usually exchange gratifications with their social workers directly as social workers get paid by society for their services. Nevertheless, clients justify the existence of social workers. But, especially following the CA, according to Sen, it is also clear that an asymmetrical distribution of power between professionals and clients or neglect of the reciprocity of perspectives endangers the necessarily participative and collaborative character of social work. For a more paternalistic approach, in contrast, this might not be a problem at all. So, in the end, it will often be inevitable to ask if a certain kind of reciprocity is compatible with the 'official' normative orientation of social work. Reciprocity could serve that way as an indicator for (in)adequate services.

Besides that, reciprocity as a moral norm might always be a challenge for social work. Due to the facts that social workers don't get gratification for their services from clients and clients are sometimes forced to use these services, it could be of added value to examine more carefully if – and to what extent – this aspect could explain failures or dysfunctionalities of social work. Because getting help without being able to return something equivalent, and being forced to become a client of social work in the first place, is a potential source of shame. Avoiding shameful situations for clients by implementing more and better opportunities for reciprocal interaction with professionals (or society) could still be an underestimated way of improving social work in general.

Conclusion

Reciprocity is indisputably a fundamental issue for social work as it determines interpersonal relations, which are constitutive of all kinds of social phenomena, including the profession itself. Therefore, an adequate assessment or understanding of social work needs to take reciprocity into account. However, the explanatory power of any kind of reciprocity and its meaning for social work depends very much on the particular normative framework of social work. Discussing the issue from the perspective of the CA illustrates this to some extent; if social work claims, e.g., to follow the CA according to Sen and fails to offer clients opportunities for (direct) reciprocal interaction, this can be seen as an indicator of an inappropriate concept of social work or – at least – as an inadequate operationalisation of the CA. According to a paternalistic interpretation of Nussbaum's CA, this would not necessarily be the case.

As a consequence, we can state that focussing more on reciprocity definitely has the potential to give us a better impression concerning the practice and the effects (representing the 'is') of social work. Furthermore, within a clear normative framework (representing the 'ought'), it should even be possible to increase this added value of reciprocity significantly. Ideally, it allows us to better assess the appropriateness of social work by comparing the observable forms of reciprocity with its self-imposed or society-predetermined normative orientation. In other words, it does not only tell us what kind of reciprocity occurs. It allows us also to ask the decisive question: if and to what extent the lack of a certain form of reciprocity actually makes sense in a given context.

Notes

1 Beings and doings that are valuable for an individual.
2 The different kinds of lives that an individual can live based on his or her resources and conversion factors.

References

Alkire, S., 2005. *Capability and Functionings: Definition & Justification*. Briefing Note. Boston, MA: Human Development and Capability Association.

Babic, B., 2011. Ohne intellektuelle Redlichkeit kein Fortschritt. Kritische Anmerkungen zum Umgang mit dem Capability Approach aus erziehungswissenschaftlicher Sicht. *In:* Sedmak, C., Babic, B., Bauer, R., and Posch, C., eds. *Der Capability Approach in sozialwissenschaftlichen Kontexten. Überlegungen zur Anschlussfähigkeit eines entwicklungspolitischen Konzepts*. Wiesbaden: VS Verlag, 75–89.

Babic, B., Eiffe, F., Gärtner, K., and Ponocny, I., eds., 2017. Well-Being -Forschung in Österreich. *Momentum Quarterly – Zeitschrift für sozialen Fortschritt* [online], 6 (2). Available from: https://www.momentum-quarterly.org/index.php/momentum.

Babic, B., Graf, G., and Germes Castro, O., 2010. The Capability Approach as a Framework for Evaluation of Child and Youth Care. *European Journal of Social Work*, 13 (3), 409–413.

Babic, B., and Leßmann, O., 2016. Zwischen Wunsch und Wirklichkeit? Schlaglichter zur Rezeption des Capability/-ies-Ansatzes in der deutschsprachigen Sozialen Arbeit. *In:* Borrmann, S., Michel-Schwartze, B., Pankofer, S., Sagebiel, J., and Spatscheck, C., eds. *Die Wissenschaft Soziale Arbeit im Diskurs - Auseinandersetzungen mit den theoriebildenden Grundlagen Sozialer Arbeit*. Opladen: Barbara Budrich, 197–216.

Becker, H., 1956. *Man in Reciprocity*. New York: Prager.

Bossong, H., 2011. Wohl-Wollen, Staatsauftrag und professionelles Eigeninteresse. Eine Kritik aktueller fachdisziplinärer Maßstäbe in der Sozialen Arbeit. *neue praxis*, 6, 591–617.

Clark, D., 2005. *The Capability Approach: Its Development, Critiques and Recent Advances*. Oxford: GPRG.

Gouldner, A., 1960. The Norm of Reciprocity: A Preliminary Statement. *American Sociological Review*, 25 (2), 161–178.

Hobhouse, L. T., 1951. *Morals in Evolution: A Study in Comparative Ethics*. London: Chapman & Hall.

Leßmann, O., Gutwald, R., and Babic, B., 2014. Der Capability-Ansatz: Ein weiterer ökonomischer Ansatz auf dem Vormarsch? *In:* Paulitzsch-Wiebe, M., Becker, B., Kunstreich, T., eds. *Politik der Sozialen Arbeit – Politik des Sozialen*. Opladen: Barbara Budrich Verlag, 160–171.

Nussbaum, M., 2000. *Women and Human Development: The Capabilities Approach*. Cambridge: Cambridge University Press.

Nussbaum, M., 2006. *Frontiers of Justice: Disability, Nationality, Species Membership*. Cambridge, MA: Harvard University Press.

OECD, ed., 2015. *How's Life? 2015: Measuring Well-Being*. Paris: OECD Publishing.

Otto, H. U., and Ziegler, H., 2006. Capabilities and Education. *Social Work & Society* [online], 4 (2), 269–287. Available from: http://www.socwork.net/sws/issue/view/10 [Accessed 13 Oct 2016].

Otto, H. U., and Ziegler, H. eds., 2012. *Das Normativitätsproblem der Sozialen Arbeit. Zur Begründung des eigenen und gesellschaftlichen Handelns.* neue praxis, Sonderheft 11, Lahnstein: Verlag neue praxis GmbH.

Perugini, M., Gallucci, M., Presaghi, F., and Ercolani, A., 2003. The Personal Norm of Reciprocity. *European Journal of Personality*, 17, 251–283.

Russel, G., 2010. In Defence of Hume's Law. *In:* Pigden, C., ed. *Hume on Is and Ought.* New York: Palgrave MacMillan, 151–161.

Scherr, A., 2012. Wieviel und welche Normativität benötigt Soziale Arbeit? *In:* Otto, H.-U. and Ziegler, H., eds. *Das Normativitätsproblem der Sozialen Arbeit. Zur Begründung des eigenen und gesellschaftlichen Handelns.* neue praxis, Sonderheft 11, Lahnstein: Verlag neue praxis GmbH, 11–24.

Schokkaert, E., 2008. *The Capabilities Approach.* Rochester, NY: Social Science Research Network.

Sen, A., 2001. *Development as Freedom.* Oxford: Oxford University Press.

Stegbauer, C., 2011. *Reziprozität. Einführung in soziale Formen der Gegenseitigkeit.* Wiesbaden: VS Verlag für Sozialwissenschaften.

Stegbauer, C., and Häußling, R., eds., 2010. *Handbuch Netzwerkforschung.* Wiesbaden: VS Verlag für Sozialwissenschaften.

Stiglitz, J., Sen, A., and Fitoussi, J. P., 2008. *Issues Paper.* Paris: Commission on the Measurement of Economic Performance and Social Progress.

Part II

Reciprocity in practice and community settings

4 Reciprocity in peer-led mutual aid groups in the community

Implications for social policy
and social work practices

Carol Munn-Giddings and Thomasina Borkman

Introduction

This chapter explores one of the fastest-growing forms of citizen-led social support networks in Europe and North America: peer-led mutual aid groups (MAGs) (Elsdon *et al.* 2000). MAGs are led and run by people with direct lived experiences of the same health conditions or social situations. We begin by defining the core characteristics and variations in practice of these groups. We identify three areas unique to MAGs that illuminate reciprocal relations: the process of the 'sharing circle,' in which peers share their own experiences and listen to those of their peers; the organisational aspects of the sharing circle; and the network of specialised relationships that evolve around the sharing circle. We explore the types of reciprocity that are manifested and embedded in these three areas and how related processes can lead to shifts in participants' understandings of their situations, increased agency and empowerment, and less stigmatised identities. Drawing on the emerging theory of relational sociology and relational social work as well as a theory of *sociality* to describe and compare differences in relationships, we illuminate the particular nature of peer-to-peer sharing and what distinguishes it from practitioner-client relations. We illustrate how MAGs are not a substitute for professional services but rather an activity that provides something that cannot be replicated in professional-client relations.

We conclude by discussing what can be learnt from this form of reciprocity and collective citizen agency and the ways in which practitioners and social policymakers can best respond to and complement citizens' own resources. In doing so, we draw particular attention to the importance of policymakers' and practitioners' understanding the difference of and distinguishing between an individual's experience of a health and social care situation and the collective knowledge and wisdom built in MAGs over time.

Definitional issues

This chapter focusses on groups of people who deliberately and voluntarily convene around a common health or social situation that is challenging and/or stigmatising for them all (thus, peers) in order to ameliorate or improve their conditions or situations. While there is great variation in the definitions of these groups and a lack of consensus in terminology, most especially within the grassroots, several academic traditions have been identified that utilise and research the same entities, irrespective of terminology used (Borkman and Munn-Giddings 2010a).

We specifically focus on groups that are peer-led, whose primary sources of knowledge about their issues are direct lived experiences, and that *predominantly occur* in the non-profit sector (Munn-Giddings *et al.* 2016). A critical feature of these groups is that they are run *for and by* the people who share the situations, which distinguishes them from groups run by trained professionals (e.g. social workers), which tend to be referred to as 'support groups' in the academic literature. MAGs are formed to change their members' situations and conditions and are not (1) social clubs whose primary interest is in socialising or other leisure time activities or (2) convened primarily as charities or philanthropies to give aid to others.

Characteristics and variations in practices of MAGs

Mutual support as voluntary action has always been part of human society in one form or another, including with Peter Kropotkin's (1914) empirical observations that mutual aid is as prevalent in the animal world as 'survival of the fittest' – a feature he theorised and applied to human societies. The form that mutual aid takes is linked to the economic, social, and political conditions in which it appears (Gidron and Chesler 1994; Dill and Coury 2008; Matzat 2010; Oka 2013).

Since the 1970s, the majority of MAGs in Europe, North and South America, and Japan have been focussed on 'single-issues' related to health or social situations. They cover every possible physical, mental health, and social condition (Munn-Giddings *et al.* 2016). They are usually instigated by an individual or a group of individuals who find they share the same situation, with a view toward supporting one another and others in the same situation. People start and join groups for a variety of reasons; whilst there is some evidence that groups start either because no service exists or because the service is inadequate or inappropriate (Borkman 1999), other research also indicates that people join who do have professional and family support but are looking for something qualitatively different, with peers who share their situations (Munn-Giddings and McVicar 2007).

Meetings are usually face-to-face whereas, as Internet usage increases, some MAGs hold 'virtual' meetings online (Boyce *et al.* 2014). Venues for meetings vary, are finance-dependent, and can include members' homes or community rooms in churches, community centres, hospitals, day centres, or libraries, among others. Many face-to-face groups meet weekly or monthly; at times, the type of condition members face (for example, Chronic Fatigue Syndrome) dictates that they meet less frequently. Meetings typically last an hour or two. Groups vary in expected duration of membership: Life transition groups (e.g. divorce, breastfeeding, or widowhood) are often short term, lasting one to two years; whereas chronic health conditions, addictions, or severe mental distress groups may be long term, lasting over decades (Borkman 1999).

As they are formed between peers, relationships are in principle egalitarian, and leadership is often rotating and ideally democratic. Help is voluntarily given without fees or money exchanges. Friendships and social relationships develop in many groups and often persist beyond participation in the group. Because they are often spontaneously organised, informal, and may have short lifespans, it is difficult to 'map' the variety and number of groups; many groups fall 'under the radar' of official statistics on voluntary action and non-profit organisations.

Internationally, MAGs vary in three important ways (Gidron and Chesler 1994):

1   Nations have varying economic, health, and welfare systems as well as civil societies, which affect the relationships between individuals, professionals, and the state;
2   Demographic, ethnic, and cultural hierarchies and variation within a country affect the kinds of relationships created; and
3   The issues and problems for which groups form affect the nature of the groups that are developed.

Important national differences have been identified: For example, in the Nordic countries with extensive health and welfare systems, many MAGs are supported by the state welfare system and can include a staff member as organiser (Stokken and Munn-Giddings 2012). In previously communist countries, such as contemporary Croatia, the state may still 'own' many health and welfare groups, including MAGs (Dill and Coury 2008). Some civil society organisations in Japan are legally required to have professional social workers provide services, thereby precluding certain kinds of peer-led mutual aid activities (Laratta 2013).

Research has also shown important differences between what are known as 12-step groups and groups that evolve more informally in the community – sometimes referred to as 'grassroots groups.' The 12-step programme, such as Alcoholics Anonymous (and the 80 other addiction and family groups patterned after AA), is primarily related to addictions and is a spiritually based programme of personal and fellowship development that involves acceptance of one's addiction and a reflexive programme of identifying one's obstacles to helping oneself and others; emphasis is placed on helping oneself by helping others – the 12th step (Riessman and Carroll 1995). These groups have networks all over the world. The 12-step groups follow organisational principles called 'traditions' of egalitarian and democratic leadership; leaders rotate and are referred to as servants of the group (Borkman 2006).

By contrast, grassroots groups that are initiated from scratch by citizens (the majority in most countries) develop their own ground rules and ways of operating – although some may be related to an overarching national charity, which may prescribe specific ways of operating. Grassroots groups may be more organisationally diverse than 12-step groups, in terms of leadership styles and reciprocity norms; groups formed by a charismatic or strong founder sometimes face succession problems (Block and Rosenburg 2002). In practice, all MAGs share some fundamental core concerns, such as space for each member to tell their story (Borkman and Munn-Giddings 2010b).

Reciprocity in MAGs' distinctive social relationships

MAGs create, utilise, maintain, comprise, and benefit from distinctive helping relationships, which are different from professional provider-service-user, volunteer-recipient, or friendship relationships (although elements of these relationships may also be present). An important part of the distinctiveness of MAG relationships is the meaning, form, and criteria of reciprocity defining them. Here, relational sociology is helpful because it describes how people's behaviour, attitudes, identity, and changes within them depend primarily on the relationships in which they are embedded and participate (Donati 2011; Burkitt 2015) and thus can illustrate and articulate MAGs' distinctive helping relationships. Relational sociology focusses on unpacking the specifics of relationships and describing and comparing in detail the elements that make them different from one another.

Alan Page Fiske (1992) has concepts of sociality that introduce and amplify differences in relationships. He delineated four elementary forms of sociality present in all cultures; we will use three of these: communal sharing, authority ranking, and equality matching. Their use will allow us to describe MAG relationships and compare them with other kinds of helping relationships, especially in terms of reciprocity behaviours. Communal sharing appears in relationships in which anyone who belongs to the designated category or group is equal to receive and give as they can; all persons are equivalent and undifferentiated. Reciprocity is defined as help that is freely given and received without calculation as to who gets how much or who gives the most. Authority ranking relationships are based on linear ordering along some hierarchical social dimension. Those higher in rank have 'prestige, prerogatives and privileges inferiors lack but subordinates are often entitled to protection and pastoral care' (Fiske 1992, p. 691). Reciprocity is defined in terms of superiors, who can appropriate or pre-empt what they wish but have some responsibility to provide for underlings. Equality matching is based on a model of even balance and one-for-one correspondence, as in turn taking, in kind reciprocity, or tit-for-tat retaliation. Each person is entitled to the same amount as other persons in the relationship, and the amounts and directions of imbalances are meaningful.

There are three areas of MAGs operation (sharing circle, organisational maintenance, and relational network) that are involved in reciprocity. The sharing circle refers to the core meeting activity of MAGs, in which members share with peers their experiences regarding the focal issues. Convening the sharing circle, other leadership functions, and associated issues of organisational maintenance are the second area. The larger network of specialised relationships and friendships that evolves around the sharing circle constitutes the third area of interest.

Fiske's three elements of sociality manifest themselves in different ways in these three areas and in MAGs with different reciprocity norms. Available research indicates that almost all MAGs operate with communal sharing in the sharing circle as discussed below. However, these insights constitute a new area of analysis, and specific research has not been done about reciprocity differences in organisational maintenance and relational networks in MAGs. It appears that a major determinant of the form of sociality (communal, hierarchical, or equality) in reciprocity involved in organisational maintenance and relational networks is the MAG's norms or lack of norms about reciprocity. When communal sharing norms are missing in organisational maintenance or in the relational network, an individual's preferences, personality, or other factors probably affect the form of sociality s/he takes, but further research is needed to clarify these areas.

Each area will be described, along with the criteria and definition of reciprocity, separately in sequence.

Sharing circle: site of communal sharing or mutual aid

The core technology of mutual aid is a process of peers sharing their own experiences and listening to others' experiences in a small group setting called a 'sharing circle,' which is inherently reciprocal. The 'sharing circle' metaphor connotes (1) the non-hierarchical and egalitarian nature of peer interaction, (2) closed and confidential participation, and (3) personal and trusting helping relationships (Borkman 1999).

In Fiske's (1992) terms, communal sharing is the basis of a MAG's sharing circle. The group develops around problem-solving a focal issue, often a chronic health problem or stigmatising social or economic issue. Anyone who faces the focal issue is usually welcome to participate and is referred to in the literature as a peer who is by definition egalitarian with fellow peers. Family members or friends of the person with the focal issue are defined differently in various groups; stroke groups include family members but separate them into different sharing circles; Alcoholics Anonymous (AA) is for alcoholics only, while family and friends convene in Al Anon groups (Borkman 1999). Professional experts in the focal issue are usually excluded from the sharing circle because they would disrupt the egalitarian interaction by introducing an element of authority ranking and threaten peer ownership of the circle. Whilst any group, including MAGs, holds the potential for power imbalances, the starting point in MAGs is that it is a relationship between peers that is interdependent rather than a relationship between someone (the professional) who doesn't share the condition but is there 'to help' others.

In the circle, individuals take turns telling some parts of their lived experiences regarding the meeting's topics. Each person's narrative about their experiences with the specific issue is somewhat different, e.g. when discussing dealing with their families' reactions to them, listeners receive various perspectives about the topic and variations in how participants handled it. According to the social theory of comparison (Brown and Lucksted 2010), participants also mentally compare themselves upwardly – e.g. if she felt better after trying that, I can try it and feel better too – and retrospectively – e.g. when I was a newcomer to the group, I made such poor decisions; I've come a long way. Members compose and relate stories or narratives about their biographies based in part on seeing their peers as role models and exemplars (Cain 1991). Hope and universality (i.e. realising one is not alone in experiencing a troublesome situation), a sense of belonging, reframing one's understanding of one's situation, and one's becoming empowered to behave and think differently are some common therapeutic factors (Kurtz 1997).

Established groups have a mixture of shorter-term and longer-term members, who have been dealing with the focal issue for some time: Some gained experiential knowledge and authority on dealing with it, and have improved their situations and outlooks, while newcomers may be upset and in early learning stages of dealing with the issue. Newcomers often arrive at MAGs in distress, having tried other means of addressing the problematic focal issue. They are greeted on a first name basis and regarded as unique whole persons (Borkman 1999), features of MAGs that signify their informality and non-bureaucratic nature. Some newcomers attend only one or two meetings and never return (Kurtz 1997). Their distress is taken seriously by the group, members of which are or have been encountering similar issues. Because they are peers with similar experiences, some can more easily identify and communicate with each other than with some other helping relationships. Others are upset to see peers with advanced conditions and leave the group. Persons whose world views or values differ from the groups' 'meaning perspectives' are unlikely to continue participation (Kurtz 1997). Persons in difficulty, precisely because of their existential suffering, become a resource for others with similar difficulties (Steinberg 1997). Individuals' weaknesses and vulnerabilities allow peers to help one another; the helper utilises his/her strengths while receiving help with his or her vulnerabilities.

Building trust between members is a fundamental building block. Megan Tschannen-Moran and Wayne K. Hoy (2000) define trust as 'one party's willingness to be vulnerable to another party based on the confidence that the latter party is: benevolent, reliable, competent, honest and open' (p. 556). Citizens who join MAGs are likely to do so when they are in a vulnerable position and when they have exhausted other forms of social support (family, friends, practitioners) or found these wanting (Munn-Giddings and

McVicar 2007). As Alan Feldman (2015) points out, if we are to proceed where there is risk, and we are vulnerable, we need to have trust in others that they will be supportive, understanding, or at least open to 'hearing' us. In MAGs, relational trust is developed through multiple means. First, individuals identify with others who have the same or similar health or social issues (Borkman 1999; Adamsen 2002). Second, the third sector setting of voluntary participation, with no required fees (and essentially free help), no bureaucracy in sight, and no professionals with superior statuses, is benevolent and monetarily non-predatory. Third, the setting is closed to non-peers and has norms of confidentiality. Only peers interact, within norms of confidentiality and with no gossiping: It is understood that what individuals say in meetings is not to be discussed with others outside it. Fourth, norms or rules about discourse that is non-judgmental, non-combative, respectful and non-patronising pertain; these norms have also been characterised as a form of dialogue (Bohm 1987, 1996; Dixon 1996). Dialogue refers to non-competitive and non-argumentative discourse in which the goal is to collectively learn and build shared understandings and system of meanings. AA and other 12-step groups evolved rules of discourse (known as no crosstalk), which include not interrupting, arguing with, or contradicting another person; speaking only from one's own experiences (self-narrative); no direct advice giving; and no discussions of politics, religion, or scientific theories (Makela *et al.* 1996, pp. 140–141). Other groups may have more conversational sharing (i.e. Sally responds directly to what Henry just said as in a conversation), but these groups are likely to have similar rules of discourse, which promote dialogue and avoid confrontation, advice giving, and discussion of politics or religion (Borkman and Munn-Giddings 2010b).

Other mechanisms strengthen reciprocity, especially humour and helping others. Humour about MAG members' situations, which would be regarded as inappropriate either in a professional setting or among non-peers, is frequently found in MAGs (Cain 1991; Munn-Giddings 2003). Making light of difficult situations is not new; Sigmund Freud (1906) discussed this as 'gallows humour,' and it is also recognised as a way of coping between professional staff in the caring professions (e.g. McCarroll *et al.* 1993; Broussine *et al.* 1999). However, in MAGs, the humour relates to a shared understanding of the seriousness of situations being faced, allowing individuals to share vulnerabilities and strengths, and enabling them to reclaim some shared 'happiness' or peace in otherwise stressful lives.

The 'sharing circle' interaction is reciprocal. On the simplest level, the presence of peers listening to others allows the circle to function and the dialogue of self-narratives to unfold, and is a form of social support per se. Within this simple interaction process, mutual help is produced; Ilkka Arminen (1998), a Finnish sociologist using conversation analysis (a methodology that analyses words, pauses, and all sentences in great detail), shows how mutual support is created by the reciprocal sharing of personal experience within a safe and trusted space in AA meetings.

Every helping relationship is in a state of imbalance, argues the psychologist Edgar Schein (2011, p. 35), with the helper being in a dominant position and the recipient or helpee in a vulnerable, dependent position. The solution to the imbalance is an intervention that builds up the helpee's status (Schein 2011, p. 47). The sharing circle provides ongoing and continuing opportunities for its members, not only to receive help but also to help others and thus keep the helper/helpee relationship in balance (as Schein recommends). Frank Riessman, an early and eminent MAG researcher, maintained that the most fundamental aspect of MAGs is that they are activities based on a form of reciprocity known as the 'helper' therapy principle. 'In its simplest form, the helper therapy principle means that those who give help are helped the most' (Riessman and Carroll 1995, p. 157). Those engaged in the group are themselves helped and enabled while helping others (Riessman 1965), and a person in difficulty, precisely because of his/her existential suffering, becomes a resource for others with similar difficulties (Steinberg 1997). Riessman (*ibid.*) argued that MAGs are so effective in part because they provide opportunities for helpees to also become helpers, that is, to play two roles of helper and helpee. Interestingly, giving help to others is often regarded by members as a major benefit of participating in MAGs (Munn-Giddings 2003; Seebohm *et al.* 2013). For example, a study of breast cancer MAGs for different ethnic/racial groups found that members in all the groups ranked 'helping others' as the greatest benefit of participating in the group, while three aspects of receiving help (learning from others, receiving encouragement, and talking about worries and fears) were ranked of lesser value (Corvin *et al.* 2013).

Organisational maintenance

A second area of reciprocity is the organisational issue of group maintenance. Within all groups, even egalitarian ones, leadership functions, such as convening the sharing circle, arranging for the venue, recruiting new members, and making coffee or tea, are needed. Large differences in the form of reciprocity in regard to organisational maintenance are found across groups, depending probably and largely on the norms of the group. Many groups rotate leadership and enlist the participation of many members in group maintenance functions – demonstrating Fiske's notion of 'communal sharing.' For example, the 12-step groups regard service to peers and to the group as a pillar of their programmes – indeed, the 12th step refers to helping peers with the programme (Makela *et al.* 1996) – thus, they have strong norms that everyone should contribute to organisational maintenance, which are norms of communal reciprocity. Seasoned members may take the lead in doing organisational tasks until newcomers are ready to help out – an example of 'serial reciprocity.'

In contrast, some or many grassroots groups do not develop norms of reciprocal obligations for how members contribute to organisational maintenance. Instead, individual leaders' preferences influence their forms of reciprocity. Louis J. Medvene and Cayla R. Teal (1997) studied grassroots groups, finding that leaders varied in their orientations to reciprocity obligations: Some individual leaders with a 'communal sharing' orientation thought reciprocity was needs-based; if an individual could or would not contribute to maintenance after receiving help from a group, it was okay. Other leaders who had an equity sharing orientation were often ambivalent about members who leave their groups after receiving what they need, without giving back to maintain the groups (Medvene and Teal 1997). In some groups, founded by forceful leaders, the founder clings to group control, thereby discouraging others from participating, which creates organisational difficulties (Block and Rosenburg 2002). Leadership in a voluntary group, in which each person is primarily there to improve his/her personal situation, can connote a function of group maintenance (Forsyth 2006) rather than directing, decision-making, or ordering people's activities. Member ownership of the group is very important for creating participation and empowering members in general and for voluntary contributions to organisational functioning; however, if no clear norms of contributing to group maintenance exist, individuals' personal definitions of what is the appropriate type of reciprocity are likely to prevail. Note that there can be tension because of differing reciprocity expectations of the 'sharing circle' and the 'organisational maintenance' functions.

Network of relationships around MAG

The third area of reciprocity is the network of relationships developed in and around the MAG. Many groups have specialised in helping relationships, such as sponsors, guides, or buddies. Sponsors in 12-step groups are seasoned members who develop a one-to-one relationship with a newcomer to guide him/her through the 12 steps and in working through the programme. Buddies join their peer in engaging in some difficult activity (e.g. members who are afraid of asserting themselves in public take a buddy to a restaurant while they practice ordering exactly what they want while stuttering (Borkman 1999). While the existence of sponsor or buddy relationships is documented in the research literature, no specific studies were found that described groups' reciprocity norms in this area in any detail. Folklore suggests that the personality of the sponsor may affect the form of sociality (Kurtz 2015). Some sponsors are described as hierarchically oriented who give orders and expect their advice to be followed without questioning; others make suggestions and discuss alternatives in a more equality ranking-like approach. Friendships also develop, in which members see each other socially outside MAG meetings, develop interpersonal closeness, and help each other as friends do; their reciprocity expectations would be personalised. Little is known about the friendships and networks created outside the circle because researchers have focussed primarily on the sharing circle and not routinely asked about outside relationships, perhaps because their research paradigm may be professional group therapy in which relationships outside the group are discouraged.

Having food, coffee, or tea, or social events alongside the circle are other mechanisms for bonding and reciprocity, but they are usually secondary to the sharing circle. Many 12-step groups celebrate individual anniversaries of sobriety with cakes, tea, and coffee. An exception to food as a secondary mechanism of bonding and reciprocity may be MAGs for self-harmers; Melanie Boyce (2016) notes that in highly stigmatised groups for self-harmers, the use of sharing and cooking food during the meeting is a way of normalising lives that are both complex and stigmatised.

The learning process, consciousness-raising, and development of agency

Participation in the sharing circle is essentially a help-receiving and help-giving learning process. The type of knowledge used and created in MAGs has been termed 'experiential knowledge,' based on direct, lived, and embodied experience; an individual's experience is subjective and may be tacit (Borkman 1976; 1999). Newcomers with new diagnoses may have little experience of their maladies. Newcomers with long-term health, economic, or social issues may have tacit knowledge and may not understand that they can know a lot from their lived experiences, but they need consciousness-raising to retrieve tacit knowledge. A reflexive process is necessary to convert 'raw experience,' which is often a jumble of inchoate images, thoughts, and feelings, into knowledge that is meaningful, with some coherence (Borkman 1976; 1999). The sharing circle provides this reflexive process, if participants engage in it. Probably, most participants, especially those who maintain membership for some time, undergo the reflexive learning process in which they gain awareness of their experiential perspective, thereby becoming empowered. Within this learning process, individuals evolve from a 'victim' stance without agency, in which they may blame others for their problems, to a 'survivor' stance in which they gain agency as actors; more advanced members can become thrivors (Borkman 1999). This consciousness-raising is empowering per se (Adamsen 2002). Seasoned members (survivors and thrivors) develop experiential authority or confidence that their experiences are valid and credible. While still peers of newcomers, the seasoned members may have more influence in the MAG because of their greater experiential authorities about ameliorating the shared condition.

MAGs are ideal exemplars of new thinking in relational sociology, in which traditional notions of structure and agency are being abandoned in favour of an analytic approach that focusses on relational connections between people, that is, '... *webs or networks of relations and interdependencies both interpersonal and impersonal, in which interactants and their joint actions are embedded'* (Burkitt 2015, p. 2). Social relationships should not be understood as merely constraining or enabling agency but as constituting the very structure and form of agency itself (*op cit*, p. 37), as is so clearly seen in MAGs.

Groups develop collective experiential knowledge and emphasise non-stigmatising approaches

Groups undergo a collective learning process over time, just as their individual members do through the 'sharing circle' (Borkman 1999). As more and more participants engage in the 'sharing circle' process, information and perspectives are accumulated, reviewed, and implicitly critiqued, which refines and deepens the experiences and knowledge about the health or social conditions that are the groups' focusses. This collective experiential knowledge is not the subjective knowledge of one person but intersubjective in that it has been accumulated and reviewed by numerous people with similar experiences, who contribute to the group because they want to improve their situations. The collective knowledge becomes more generalised and universalised information as more members with varying backgrounds and experiences contribute to it (Adamsen 2002).

Many MAGs reject part or all of the mainstream and conventional biomedical or other professional perspectives on their issues and develop their own alternative 'meaning perspectives' (Borkman and Munn-Giddings 2008). Thomasina Borkman (1999) identified the viewpoints about the focal issue and its amelioration or improvement as 'meaning perspectives'; she called significantly alternative world views or perspectives of an issue that challenge mainstream and biomedical/professional perspectives 'liberating meaning perspectives.'

MAGs for short-term conditions or life transitions seem to be primarily for social support and coping with a troublesome situation, and to utilise simple common-sense coping and support strategies. In contrast, some groups for chronic or long-term conditions, such as severe mental health problems or addictions, develop elaborate and codified programmes of individual change and identity transformation, which also tend to be 'liberating meaning perspectives'; these include the 12-step programmes for the eighty or more anonymous addiction and associated family groups and three MAGs for serious and persistent mental health problems. MAGs for mental health problems with transformative programmes include (1) GROW, based on an adaptation of the 12 steps (Rappaport 1993); (2) Recovery International (previously Recovery, Inc.; see Kurtz 2015); and (3) the Hearing Voices Network (Noorani 2012). The latter two developed codified programmes without adopting the 12 steps. With GROW (which originated in Australia and spread to the U.S.) and Recovery International (which originated in the U.S.), individuals whose lives and identities were limited to identities as mental health patients with all the implied stigma develop constructive new identities as ordinary members of a 'caring and sharing' community (and part-time incidental patients of the mental health system) (Rappaport 1993). In the Hearing Voices Movement (which originated in the Netherlands but is now in twenty-nine countries worldwide), individuals have developed a programme to learn to understand and live with their voices in a constructive way instead of trying to remove the voices, as is the goal of the biomedical model (Noorani 2012); many of them leave limited roles as mental health patients for wider roles as citizens in the community, similar to GROW and Recovery International members.

In the 12-step addiction groups, successful members undergo a conversion or transformation process over time from non-productive and stigmatised 'drunk' or drug addict identities to those of abstinent and productive recovering alcoholics or drug addicts (Cain 1991; Denzin 1993). The anonymity of the programmes may result in the sources of their changes being unknown to the outside world.

Whether the MAG employs simple common-sense coping strategies or has elaborated programmes of individual change and identity transformation, they generally find ways to understand and live with their situations as part of being human in normalising and non-stigmatising ways. A major point of contrast between MAGs and professional, biomedical, and mainstream theories is that the latter tend to emphasise diagnoses and pathologies and how to eradicate them instead of how to constructively live with them, which is the focus of MAGs. Matthew E. Archibald (2007, p. 10) regards the mutual aid social movement as a 'collective challenge to constituted authority in nongovernmental institutional domains.'

In conclusion, reciprocity in the form of mutual aid is different from the help received by service-users/clients from professionals. When professionals lead support groups, and peers do not own and control the group, the professionals' authority rankings (Fiske 1992) are likely to dampen the communal sharing and reciprocity found in MAGs. It is likely that help-giving opportunities will be minimised, fewer relationships outside the group will evolve, and the professionals' 'meaning perspectives' will dominate the groups (Chesler and Cheney 1995; Borkman 1999; Oka 2013).

Conflict and other negative aspects of MAGs

MAGs, like all small groups, can experience conflict over such issues as 'meaning perspectives,' leadership, group procedures, or domineering or disruptive members (Chesler 1990; Forsyth 2006; Borkman 2016). In the early days of MAGs, some professionals thought they could be 'dangerous' to lay members because they would spread misinformation, create emotional problems for members, or harbour troubled people who need specialised professional attention; these and other possible 'dangers' have not been substantiated to any extent by research (Chesler 1990; Borkman 2016). MAGs readily acknowledge that they cannot help and do not want to try to help severely troubled individuals and report asking such people to seek specialised professional help (Borkman 2016).

A major escape valve for avoiding conflict in groups is their voluntary and small group nature. People who do not like the direction of a group will vote with their feet, so to speak, and stop attending. Groups with extensive leadership problems, continuing conflict over procedures or 'meaning perspectives,' or the inability to contain disruptive members are likely to self-destruct, disband, or wither away for lack of attendance. New groups are relatively easy to initiate, with some exceptions, such as in Japan (Oka 2003). There is a saying in 12-step groups that all you need to start a new group are two people with a resentment and a coffee pot. Starting new groups is very likely, except in rural areas or for relatively rare conditions, which may mean that there may be too few potential members. However, with extensive internet, capabilities in most areas online groups can be created.

Discussion: what can we learn from MAGs? Implications for policy and practice

In recent years, a number of health and social care policies in Europe and North America have begun to encroach on areas traditionally occupied by MAGs, including, for example, social policies related to Self-Care, Expert Patient Programme, and the move towards increasing choice through personal budgets for health and social care needs. Support for 'mutual aid' is advocated from a variety of conflicting standpoints, including genuine responses to service-users' assuming more control over their lives as well as from neoliberal austerity policies and their consequent impact on reducing mainstream professional services. Equally, there is an increasing interest in the use of experiential knowledge to inform services and 'peer-led' schemes, although the latter tend to be dominated by individualistic models of practice through one-to-one peer support schemes and workers (Boyce 2016).

Professionals and policymakers tend to underestimate or be unaware of the difference between an individual's experience of a health or social condition and the collective knowledge of established MAGs. Yet it is crucial in understanding how some groups have come to redefine their situations or conditions with their 'liberating meaning perspectives.' Further, the difference between an individual service-user/patient with a diagnosis and corresponding status, such as breast cancer patient, and a seasoned MAG member, with experiential authority of his/her condition, is often not recognised or appreciated by professionals or policymakers (Munn-Giddings 2003; Boyce 2016). Many countries have policies that promote the involvement of 'experts by experience' (people with a direct experience of a health condition) in service development and delivery, but often, professionals and policymakers select an individual with a given status (i.e. diagnosis or type of service-user) to represent a given category to fulfil their quotas of service-user participation instead of inviting a member from a mature MAG with collectivised knowledge of the condition to give their views (Munn-Giddings 2003). The only exception we know of is Germany, which has a system to ensure that experientially knowledgeable people are selected to represent their disease/condition categories by ensuring that health providers work first and foremost with established MAGs that have collectivised experiential knowledge of their members (Matzat 2010).

The mutual aid ethos of voluntarily and freely given help within egalitarian and communal peer sharing relationships is so central to groups and is both strong and vulnerable at the same time. If health and social care policymakers and professionals fail to grasp the fundamental nature and ethos of peer-led MAGs, they could damage or undermine their very essence. A fundamental question therefore is: What lessons can we learn from citizens' own agency and the reciprocal processes they have pioneered to inform policy and practice developments?

There are at least three critical features of peer-led MAGs that it is important for policymakers and practitioners to understand and learn from. Peer-led MAGs offer something quite unique in terms of their *social relations, processes,* and the ensuing *collective knowledge* base that is built through the sharing circle. Taken together, these are the building blocks for a form of collective agency. As Ian Burkitt (2015) posits, the concept of agency in social theory (to which we might add social policy and social work) changes when it is conceptualised as a *relational* rather than an *individual* phenomenon. Contrary to the ideals of mainstream Western moral and political thought, which celebrate individuality, independence, and autonomy as primary goals for citizens, MAGs offer us a vision in which agency emerges and is enacted through the sharing of vulnerabilities as well as strengths, and the resulting interdependence is by definition reciprocal.

New directions in relational social work (Donati 2011) also offer opportunities for exploring how practitioners can co-construct the helping process for the well-being of service-users and practitioners alike. Relational social work focusses on relationships as the basis for change – a practice paradigm in which practitioners identify and resolve problems by facilitating coping networks (conceived as a set of relationships between people interested in a common aim) to enhance resilience and capacities for action at both an individual and collective level (Raineri and Cabiati 2015, p. 2). Central to the philosophy and practice is that change emerges from reciprocal aid, between both the social worker and people in difficult circumstances, family members, friends, neighbours, and other networks. The role of the practitioner is therefore that of the enabler, who helps the network develop reflexivity and improve itself in enhancing welfare. In turn, the network helps the practitioner to better understand how s/he can help (Folgheraiter and Raineri 2012). MAGs form an important part of many service-users' support networks – grasping the importance of this moves social work and policy from an individualistic model to one that acknowledges and encompasses the collective.

Importantly, MAGs are not a substitute for professional services but rather an activity that provides something that cannot be replicated in professional-client relations. Their uniqueness resides in the experiential knowledge; peer-helping social relations; and special, non-hierarchical communal sharing processes of these groups. Sometimes, the knowledge generated within them challenges our preconceptions of a health condition or problem situation. At other times, such knowledge can complement and inform professional service development.

Policies that support the facilitative infrastructures and practices of MAGs are key. Examples include policies that support clearing houses that link groups and provide them with resources to nurture MAGs. Equally, facilitative and sensitive practitioners can help MAGs to blossom. Practices that begin from the standpoint of enablement and mutual respect lead to a variety of enabling roles, which usefully support rather than intervene in MAGs (Wilson 1995; ESTEEM 2013; Munn-Giddings *et al.* 2017). A helpful theoretical discussion by Tomofumi Oka and Thomasina Borkman identifies the role social workers could have with MAGs as a 'mutual aid supporter,' that is, as professionals, officials, or anyone who is not a peer member of a group but who '*respects the autonomy and integrity of the group and works as the members wish*' (2011, p. 16).

One of the functions of relational social work consists of creating the conditions for mutual aid through a style of intervention that favours empowerment, conceiving of client 'problems' not as pathologically driven but rather as difficulties in social coping with life tasks; this shifts the problem from the person to the assistance required, and the social worker's role moves from someone whose intervenes and addresses 'problems' to a facilitator of citizens' own agencies and resources at the individual and collective level.

In this chapter, we have outlined the ways in which citizens themselves develop mutual aid in MAGs through the sharing circle and by illuminating their core forms of reciprocity. It should be noted that in this form of citizen reciprocity, informality is both a strength and weakness – the unique form of social relations that being a 'peer' (rather than client or service-user) generates thus produces the conditions for mutual aid, such as the common purpose, the identification with one another, and the members' being motivated by distress to change their lives and in doing so help others. However, interventionist rather than facilitative practices and policies can easily undermine the ethos of mutuality. Therefore, understanding and appreciating the practices in MAGs offers learning opportunities for social workers and policymakers in relation to their role(s) in supporting a welfare landscape that values the strengths and capabilities of both individuals and collectives of citizens.

References

Adamsen, L. 2002. 'From victim to agent': The clinical and social significance of self-help group participation for people with life-threatening diseases. *Scandinavian Journal of Caring Sciences*, 16, 224–231.

Archibald, M. E. 2007. *The Evolution of self-help: How a health movement became an institution.* New York: Palgrave Macmillan.

Arminen, I. 1998. *Therapeutic interaction: A study of mutual help in the meetings of alcoholics anonymous.* Helsinki: The Finnish Foundation for Alcohol Studies.

Block, S. R. and Rosenburg, S. 2002. Toward an understanding of founder's syndrome: An assessment of power and privilege among founders of nonprofit organizations. *Nonprofit Management and Leadership,* 12, 352–368.

Bohm, D. 1987. *Unfolding meaning.* London: Routledge.

Bohm, D. 1996. *On dialogue.* London: Routledge.

Borkman, T. 1976. Experiential knowledge: A new concept for the analysis of self-help group. *Social Service Review,* 50 (September), 445–456.

Borkman, T. 1999. *Understanding self-help/mutual aid: Experiential learning in the commons.* New Brunswick, NJ: Rutgers University Press.

Borkman, T. 2006. Sharing experience, conveying hope: Egalitarian relations as the essential method of alcoholic anonymous. *Nonprofit Management and Leadership,* 17 (3), 145–161.

Borkman, T. 2016. Conflict in self-help/mutual aid groups. Unpublished paper. Silver Spring, MD.

Borkman T. and Munn-Giddings, C. 2008. Self-help groups challenge health care systems in the US and UK. In: Chambre S. and Goldner, M., (Eds.) *Patients, Consumers and Civil Society: US and International Perspectives,* Vol. 10 Advances in Medical Sociology. Emerald Group Publishing; Bingley, UK, 127–150.

Borkman, T. and Munn-Giddings, C. 2010a. Different traditions of self-help/mutual aid research: Their contribution to developing third sector knowledge. Paper presented at 9th Conference of ISTR, Kadir Has University, Istanbul, Turkey, July 7–10.

Borkman, T. and Munn-Giddings, C. 2010b. Talk in carers' and alcoholics anonymous self-help group meetings. Unpublished paper.

Boyce, M. 2016. It's a safe space: The role of self-harm self-help/mutual aid groups. PhD Thesis. Chelmsford (UK): Anglia Ruskin University.

Boyce, M., Munn-Giddings, C., Seebohm, P., Chaudary, S. and Avis, M. 2014. Use of social media by self-help/mutual aid groups. *Groupwork,* 24 (2), 26–44.

Broussine, M., Davies, F. and Calvert Scott, J., 1999. Humour at the edge: An inquiry into the use of humour in British social work at: http://www.uwe.ac.uk/bbs/trr/Issue1/IS1-2_1.htm.

Brown, L. and Lucksted, A. 2010. Theoretical foundations of mental health self-help. In: Louis D. Brown and Scott Wituk, (Eds.) *Mental Health Self-Help: Consumer and Family Initiatives.* NY: Springer Science + Business Media, LLC, 19–38.

Burkitt, I. 2015. Relational agency: Relational sociology, agency and interaction. *European Journal of Social Theory,* 1–18.

Cain, C. 1991. Personal stories: Identity acquisition and self understanding in alcoholics anonymous. *Ethos,* 19 (2), 210–253.

Chesler, M. A. 1990. The "dangers" of self-help groups: Understanding and challenging professionals' views. In: Powell, T. J., (Ed.) *Working with Self-Help.* Silver Spring, MD: National Association of Social Workers, 301–324.

Chesler, M. A. and Chesney, B. K. 1995. *Cancer and self-help: Bridging the troubled waters of childhood illness.* Madison, WI: University of Wisconsin Press.

Corvin, J., Coreil, J., Nupp, R. and Dyer, K. 2013. Ethnic differences in cultural models of breast cancer support groups. *International Journal of Self-Help and Self Care,* 7 (2), 193–215.

Denzin, N. K. 1993. *The alcoholic society: Addiction and recovery of the self.* New Brunswick, NJ: Transaction Publishers.

Dill, A. and Coury, J. 2008. Forging a new commons: Self help associations in Slovenia and Croatia. In: Chambre S. and Goldner, M., (eds.) *Patients, Consumers and Civil Society: US and International Perspectives*, Vol. 10 Advances in Medical Sociology. Bingley: Emerald Group Publishing.

Dixon, N. M. 1996. *Perspectives on dialogue: Making talk developmental for individuals and organizations.* Greensboro, NC: Center for Creative Leadership.

Donati, P., 2011. *Relational sociology: A new paradigm for the social sciences.* London: Routledge.

Elsdon, K., Reynolds, J. and Stewart, S., 2000. *Sharing experience, living and learning: A study of self-help groups.* London: Community Matters.

ESTEEM. 2013. Project summaries and resources available at Self Help Nottingham: Retrieved January 6, 2016 from: http://www.selfhelp.org.uk/research/.

Feldman, A. 2015. *Trust in action research.* Presentation at the annual meeting of the Collaborative Action Research Network, Braga, Portugal, November 6–8, November 2.

Fiske, A. P. 1992. The four elementary forms of sociality: Framework for a unified theory of social relations. *Psychological Review*, 99 (4), 689–723.

Folgheraiter, F. and Raineri, M. L. 2012. A critical analysis of the social work definition according to the relational paradigm. *International Social Work*, 55, 473–487.

Forsyth, D. R. 2006. *Group dynamics.* 4th Edition. Belmont, CA: Thomson Wadsworth.

Freud, S. 1906. *Jokes and their relation to the unconscious.* New York: Norton.

Gidron, B. and Chesler, M. 1994. Universal and particular attributes of self-help: A framework for international and intranational analysis. *Prevention in Human Services*, 11 (1), 1–44.

Kropotkin, P. 1914. *Mutual aid: A factor in evolution.* Boston, MA: Porter Sargent.

Kurtz, L. F. 1997. *Self-help and support groups: A handbook for practitioners.* Thousand Oaks, CA: Sage Publications.

Kurtz, L. F. 2015. *Recovery groups: A guide to creating, leading, and working with groups for addictions and mental health conditions.* New York: Oxford University Press.

Laratta, R. 2013. A study in accountability of clubhouses in Japan, UK, and Italy. *International Journal of Self-Help and Self-Care*, 7 (1), 81–97.

Makela, K. et al. 1996. *Alcoholics anonymous as a mutual-help movement: A study in eight societies.* Madison, WI: University of Wisconsin Press.

Matzat, J. 2010. Self-help/mutual aid in Germany: A 30 year perspective of a participant observer. *International Journal of Self-Help and Self Care*, 5 (3), 279–294.

McCarroll, J. E., URJ., Wright, K. M. and Fullerton, C. S. 1993. Handling bodies after violent death: Strategies for coping. *American Journal of Orthopsychiatry*, 63 (2) April 2, 09–214.

Medvene, L. J. and Teal, C. R. 1997. Leaders' ambivalence about reciprocity obligations in self-help groups. *Small Group Research*, 28 (2), 302–322.

Munn-Giddings, C. 2003. *Mutuality and movement: An exploration of the relationship of self help/mutual aid to social policy.* Ph.D. dissertation, Department of Social Policy, Loughborough University, Loughborough, UK.

Munn-Giddings, C., Avis, M., Boyce, M., Chaudhary, S. and Seebohm, P. 2017. Being a 'self-help supporter': Recognising the roles that community practitioners can adopt in supporting self-help groups. *Research, Policy and Planning*, 32 (2), 113–125.

Munn-Giddings, C. and McVicar, A. 2007. Self-help groups as mutual support: What do carers value? *Health and Social Care in the Community*, 15 (1), 26–34.

Munn-Giddings, C., Oka, T., Borkman, T., Matzat, J., Montano, R. and Chikot, G. 2016. Self-help and mutual aid group volunteering. In: Horton-Smith and Grotz, (eds.) *Palgrave Research Handbook of Volunteering and Non-profit Associations.*

Noorani, T. 2012. Self-help expertise and spinoza: Re-imagining capacities within the mental health service user/survivor movement, unpublished PhD dissertation, University of Bristol, UK.

Oka, T. 2003. Self-help groups for parents of children with intractable diseases: A qualitative study of their organisational problems. Parkland, FL.Dissertation. com.

Oka, T. 2013. Grief is love: Understanding grief through self-help groups organised by the family survivors of suicide. In: Drautzburg, A. A. and Oldfield, J. (Eds.) *Making Sense of Suffering: A Collective Attempt.* Freeland, Oxfordshire, UK: Inter-Disciplinary Press, 75–86.

Oka, T. and Borkman, T. 2011. SHGs, self-help supporters and social work: a theoretical discussion with some case illustrations of family survivors of suicide in Japan. *Studies on Social Work*, 37 (3), 168–183.

Raineri, M. L. and Cabiati, E. 2015. Kitwood's thought and relational social work. *European Journal of Social Work*. doi: 10.1080/13691457.2015.1074549.

Rappaport, J. 1993. Narrative studies, personal stories, and identity transformation in the mutual help context. *Journal of Applied Behavioral Science*, 29, 230–256.

Riessman, F. 1965. The 'helper' therapy principle. *Social Work*, 10 (2), 27–32.

Riessman, F. and Carroll, D. 1995. *Redefining self-help: policy and practice.* San Francisco, CA: Jossey-Bass, Inc. Publishers.

Schein, E. H. 2011. *Helping: How to offer, give, and receive help.* San Francisco, CA: Brett-Koehler Publishers.

Seebohm, P., Boyce, M., Chaudhary, S., Avis, M. and Munn-Giddings, C. 2013. The contribution of self-help/mutual aid groups to mental wellbeing. *Health and Social Care in the Community*, 21 (4), 391–401.

Steinberg, D. M., 1997. *The mutual aid approach to working with groups: Helping people help each other.* New York: Aronson.

Stokken, R. and Munn-Giddings, C. 2012. Self-help/mutual aid in Nordic countries: Introduction to the special Nordic issue. *International Journal of Self Help and Self Care*, 6 (1), 3–9.

Tschannen-Moran, M. and Hoy, W. K. 2000. A multidisciplinary analysis of the nature, meaning, and measurement of trust. *Review of Educational Research, 70* (4), 547–593.

Wilson, J. 1995. *Two worlds: Self help groups and professionals.* Birmingham: British Association of Social Workers.

5   Revisions to client and professional self-categorisations during reciprocal support groups among the long-term unemployed in Finland

Laura Tarkiainen

Introduction

In this chapter, I aim to illustrate what kinds of revised self-categorisations long-term unemployed clients and the professionals working with them re-craft whilst sharing their experiences through open-ended interviews among support groups. At a wider contextual level, this chapter also presents a discussion of the importance of understanding the unique role and potential of group engagement as a reciprocally oriented social work practice. I conceptualise reciprocity as a general intention to give as well as receive in life – rather than an expectation of a tit-for-tat mutual exchange – as well as a sense of 'usefulness' to other individuals, communities or society in general (see Thompson 2013, xiii).

My analysis focusses on data collected during 15 group interviews amongst 65 long-term unemployed adults and four group interviews amongst 16 professionals who work with them. The majority of unemployed adults interviewed – whom I refer to as clients – faced multiple barriers related to their employability. These included a range of limitations, such as mental health issues, substance abuse, low education levels and complex social circumstances, all of which hampered their abilities to immediately sustain paid work. Prior to the interviews, clients voluntarily attended a support group aimed at helping them to better balance their daily lives and to generally improve their health and well-being through support from their peers and empathetic professionals in their local communities.

My analysis should be understood within a specific context. Thus, I first describe the wider social, cultural, political and institutional landscape within which my interviewees' experiences emerged and in which they are situated. I pay particular attention to the role of welfare institutions in conveying various negative and stigmatising categories as well as the reciprocal dynamics of category formation. From my research, I find that social work and welfare structures play a key role in producing and reshaping clients' self-perceptions through categorisation. Instead of being categorised by the welfare system, social work clients – particularly those with prolonged unemployment histories – may benefit from real opportunities to create new and empowering self-categorisations and positive views of themselves. This may be achieved through voicing and sharing their experiences in different group settings where alternative self-categorisations are reciprocally produced and constructed, both in client-to-client and client-to-professional relationships.

Finnish unemployment services processing of its unemployed clients

In unemployment research, the concept of reciprocity is often discussed in relation to the rights and duties of the citizen and the state. Different welfare regimes hold varying expectations of what it means to be a 'deserving' citizen and to what extent reciprocity is incorporated into prevailing norms about socially valued and expected behaviour. The Finnish social democratic welfare regime is based on the idea that 'everybody gives to everybody,' therefore determining if recipients of benefits and services have reciprocated remains difficult (Larsen 2006). Yet in selective welfare models, systemic reciprocity is perceived as being very low, which increases the importance of grateful and compliant attitudes among those receiving targeted benefits and services (*ibid.*).

Over the last decade, however, the Finnish welfare system has steadily moved towards the idea of active citizenship as its ideal, highlighting an obligation to work and an individual's responsibility, and amplifying the conditionality of welfare assistance (Keskitalo 2008). In the obligating approach, the state asks citizens to more actively fulfil their duties – such as taking part in various programmes – in return for social benefits and welfare support (see Kjørstad 2016). These policies focus on promoting self-reliance, even amongst individuals facing major social and health barriers to entering the labour market (Keskitalo 2008, Närhi and Kokkonen 2014).

Thus, similar to situations in several other welfare states, municipal social workers assume a key role in 'activating' the unemployed clients in Finland (Kroll and Blomberg 2011). Therefore, a central goal of social work lies in transforming its unemployed clients into something else (Mäkitalo and Säljö 2002a). In other words, social workers' transformative tasks aim at encouraging clients to construct identities that in one way or another relate to the labour market (Caswell *et al.* 2011). This means that social work's institutional practices consist of systematic attempts to produce certain kinds of people with appropriate self-perceptions by categorising them (Mäkitalo and Säljö 2002b) in order to promote and locally govern various social and labour market policies.

In Finland, social work amongst long-term unemployed clients primarily proceeds through individualised approaches. That is, social work aims to solve social problems separately for each individual, with a weak tradition of group or community-based approaches to service selection (Roivainen 2009). In particular, the culturally predominant bureaucratic adult social work carried out amongst long-term unemployed clients is at risk of narrowing its focus to a profession of control whereby clients are defined as dependent and passive objects of work (Juhila *et al.* 2003).

Paradoxically, as Vappu Karjalainen (2014) states, those most in need receive little if any institutional attention within the Finnish welfare system because institutions primarily focus on preventing individuals from becoming long-term unemployed. Some unemployed individuals are categorised as 'hopeless cases' or 'too hard to help.' That is, welfare system providers perceive them as unlikely to obtain steady employment and, therefore, provide little or inadequate support to them. In turn, those categorised as employable are targeted earlier and perceived as clients who are 'good and easy to work with.'

However, clients are not just passive participants upon whom categories are forced by institutions and social workers but active participants resisting and sometimes avoiding labour market-oriented identities and categories offered by the welfare system (Caswell *et al.* 2011, Tarkiainen 2017). Therefore, categorisations are not only forced upon the client but rather reciprocally negotiated and co-constructed, for example, in collaboration between the client and the social worker (Juhila and Abrams 2011, Juhila *et al.* 2014). Thus, in welfare practices, individuals are both constructed and engaged in constructing their own identities (see Fook 2002, p. 76, 89).

Categorisation within social work focusses on identifying clients' problems and fostering and stimulating specific capacities in a way that renders problems manageable by and within the system (Caswell *et al.* 2011). In this sense, social work performs as a profession that processes clients in order to place them into predetermined slots within an institution's classification system and stimulates clients to assess themselves in such terms (Hjörne *et al.* 2010). Thus, various competing consequential categorisations related to class, health and social problems exist within social work (Juhila and Abrams 2011).

Categorisation in social work is an extremely delicate task because assigning individuals to specific categories creates identities. Thus, how individuals are identified, categorised and labelled by others shapes their self-identifications. Therefore, social workers must be particularly conscious of their participation in categorising that produces, maintains, modifies and brokers identities. In turn, these are produced and redefined within reciprocal encounters and governed by larger welfare policies and discourses (Juhila *et al.* 2003, Juhila and Abrams 2011).

Study aims, data and methods

My data is drawn from the three-year Rytmi Project (2009–2011) funded by the European Social Fund. This project aimed to improve and support the health and everyday well-being of unemployed individuals. These individuals held a weak labour market position, residing in small- and medium-sized

Finnish towns in the rural and urban areas of the Päijät-Häme and Itä-Uusimaa regions. To achieve these objectives, the project assisted local social and health service providers to implement a service path including physical health examinations and support groups, into existing local service structures.

Local unemployed individuals were reached via social services or local employment offices. Then, providers offered them an optional health examination and the opportunity to voluntarily take part in a professionally led, face-to-face support group that met eight times over a three- to five-month period, depending on the group. Participants had prolonged unemployment histories, and most held somewhat limited work abilities. For my study, I defined long-term unemployment as being unemployed for one year or more.

Group meetings thematically focussed on various mundane practices, such as participants' habits and routines around diet, sleep, exercise and socialising as these were embedded in their daily lives. These everyday practices were discussed and reflected upon through various group discussions and written assignments, both during and outside the group (e.g. diary methods mapped the daily routines and happenings of each participant). In addition, group participants were offered the opportunity to meet with a dietitian, while other collaborating municipalities offered group participants additional services, such as free access to local sports centres. Support groups also aimed to engage community members in various activities and interactions in order to address shared concerns.

In groups, each member was asked to set an individual midterm and easy-to-achieve lifestyle change, embedded in their everyday activities and routines, such as restructuring daily schedules, moderately reducing alcohol consumption or meeting friends on a regular basis. The core idea of the support group focussed on activating and empowering the everyday lives of individuals with the help of peers and professionals. This was achieved through gradual progress towards regaining balance in clients' everyday lives rather than immediately aiming for them to return to work. Professionals were trained to lead support groups with goal-oriented and empowering methods, which did not explicitly focus on reciprocity or mutual aid.

Most participants needed rehabilitative services prior to gaining employment, while some, in fact, perceived themselves as unemployable (see Tarkiainen 2017). Participants represented a heterogeneous group in terms of age, gender, educational attainment and employment histories, yet most shared a low level of education and sporadic work histories. Wishes to engage in meaningful activities during the day, to meet peers and to make level-headed changes in their lives were identified as reasons to participate in the group.

Two pilot studies were conducted within the larger project in order to localise solid support group practices, which were then related to the existing service structures. In the project, an action-research approach and the 'User Participation in Quality Assessment' (Krogstrup 1997) method was used to collect, analyse and report data. In keeping with the action-research method, both clients and professionals played a key role in improving the services at hand and were, therefore, interviewed. All face-to-face interviews were carried out in various institutional settings where groups normally gathered, such as in social service and rehabilitative units and local community centres. Three project members conducted the interviews, including myself.

Prior to the interviews, interviewers observed the last support group meeting after permission was granted in order to gain insight into each group. Each group had three to eight participants, and almost all participants were interviewed, excluding those who dropped out (around one-fifth of all participants). One limitation to this data set lies in the lack of interviews among dropouts; most likely, the group interview dynamics influenced the ways that interviewees shared their thoughts. Thus, the pitfalls, complexities and critical voices regarding the support group experiences remained mostly silent.

Each interview lasted approximately one to two hours. Client interview questions focussed on participants' experiences within the support group they attended as well as their previous experiences as service-users. During the interviews, we asked participants how the support group model could be improved, to identify the benefits and weaknesses of the group and how this group compared to previous service experiences that they had as unemployed service-users. In addition, we were interested in the professionals' experiences. After organising 15 group interviews among clients between 2010 and 2011, we conducted four group interviews among 16 professionals in 2011. Professionals represented health, social work and rehabilitation service providers.

The local ethics committee approved the project's study, whereby the study and data collection met all ethical principles, such as confidentiality and the possibility of withdrawing from the study. During all interviews, we used a semi-structured interview guide, whereby the open-ended questions posed depended on how each interview evolved. Each participant signed an informed consent form prior to the interview, and all interviews were audio-taped and then transcribed to text, resulting in 350 pages of client interview data and 85 pages of professional interview data. Interviews were conducted in Finnish, while excerpts were translated into English.

Furthermore, the interviews were not specifically on self-categorisations nor on reciprocity; however, I obtained permission to use the data collected during the project for my own analysis. In this, I focussed on the revised self-categorisations posed by interviewees, despite my awareness that the interview situation itself influenced self-categorisations. In my analysis, I ask,

What kinds of revised self-categorisations do long-term unemployed clients and professionals working in unemployment services create through their discourse when they share their experiences within a support group?

Here, I focus on the revised self-categorisations that emerged in the discourse during interviews and seek to identify in what ways interviewees self-categorise. In my analysis, I first read through the data in its entirety several times and coded it inductively, thereafter rereading it. When sifting through the data, I tracked the revised self-categorisations, both in client and professional interviews, reading through the transcripts again and specifically focussing on those revisions. Subsequently, I focussed on extracts from my data dealing with self-categorisations and mapped them according to the key recurring themes that emerged during the interviews. As a result of my analysis, I grouped five self-categorisations under the themes of *revised client categorisations* and *revised professional categorisations*. In what follows, I use ten excerpts from the interviews to illustrate various points in my analysis.

Revised client categorisations

First, in my analysis, I focus on clients' revised self-categorisations, which I have identified as follows: *'active life changer'*, *'supporter'* and *'equally encountered'*.

Active life changer

In my data analysis, I noticed that clients included extensive descriptions of re-examining their prior selves and envisioning future potential alternative self-categorisations. For example, individuals expressed some hope as they potentially moved closer to becoming fit for work and living a stable and active life:

> I think this group has been a great experience. These meetings and all these people I got to know have been wonderful. When I was just at home, I did nothing but sit at the computer, going to the fridge and lazing on the sofa. Now, because of this group, I gained some ideas of how to change my own life and I can now see, that, wow, things can go this other way as well. This has had a real influence on me. Outside this group some of us have started to take walks together and those walks have been huge sources of supports to me as well. We can catch up and share our experiences and thoughts, which has been really important.
>
> (Client interview 1)

This interviewee categorised herself as being an *'active life changer'* as opposed to the *'passive layabout'* she had felt she was previously. In this way, the interviewee moved beyond the negative unemployment identity and formed her own more positive self-image. Her revision of her self-categorisation is visible in the way she describes herself – feeling engaged, supported and living an active life.

During the interviews, clients repeatedly argued against the dehumanising classification mechanisms embedded in the service system for Finland's unemployed. In particular, the support group's focus on mundane habits and improving everyday life proved appealing, ultimately prompting attendance. However, for many clients, simply having the courage to take part in and commit to the support group represented a significant achievement. In the excerpt below, one interviewee discussed why he previously avoided peer and support groups and why he now chose to take part:

> I have never been a group-spirited person really – never previously considered peer groups. Let's say groups like Alcoholics Anonymous must have a good atmosphere, but it only involves sharing what happened and how much I've drunk and never focuses on describing your good sides and describing me as a human being. You don't really get to know yourself when you always tell the same story about being 14 and waking up in a ditch and the police picking me up. So, you sort of tell the same story over and over again, and it doesn't really move on from there. Then, I came to this group, because I need to improve my everyday life for myself and my health. Even small things are big things – a change and improvement for the better. Like having a hangover just once a month is already a big change for me. So, through this group, I sort of woke up that, damn it, does it have to be like this? I've been asked to take part in a community centre in my neighbourhood. They have all kinds of activities, so I could participate and change. It's only 100 metres away from my place. I could go there when they meet. There are all kinds of people, playing cards and doing all kinds of things. Anyway, by going, I could change my life a bit, because sometimes my life is bloody depressing.
>
> (Client interview 2)

In the above extract, the interviewee defines himself by using the alcoholic category but seeks to view his problematic alcohol consumption as a part of his ordinary everyday life, which also featured some good elements and positive characteristics. The interviewee looks at his *'depressing life'* from a different perspective after attending the group, which also renders him as a potential *'life changer'*.

In addition, the interviewee recounts how he avoided peer support groups because he wanted to be seen beyond the category of alcoholic – in other words, as a human being. Previously, he was not motivated to attend any groups because he thought the problem category labels explicitly lay at the centre of the groups' attention. According to the client, peer and support groups based on problem categories encourage the internalisation of a deviant category, whilst other more positive self-categorisations remain easily submerged.

Many clients highlighted the importance of the group's holistic approach and focus on everyday life, which takes into account the humanness of all participants. Furthermore, the group's approach, to a certain extent, invalidated the categorical labels often used in various individual and group-based social work practices, such as alcoholic, mentally ill and the long-term unemployed.

Supporter

According to clients, opportunities for reciprocity created through sharing experiences strengthened their senses of normalcy and belonging whilst diminishing their feelings of being less valuable in comparison to others. Clients described a variety of reciprocal helping processes between support group members by categorising themselves as holding dual roles, that is, as people who receive but also provide support. Below, one interviewee describes his own self-image as somehow inadequate and devalued in his own and others' eyes before he attended the support group:

> For me, in this group, I realised that I am not the only one who struggles with these issues. I thought I was alone in this community. But, there are other people as well who have some difficulties. It has helped me a lot to move forward. It has made me feel better, and now I do not always blame myself and feel guilty. I am not always the only one to blame. I have realised that there are others who go through the same thing and who have their own problems. While we don't really know each other, we've been able to speak about our issues. And, funnily, it has helped me, since I've been able to help other people and been able to speak.
>
> (Client interview 3)

As shown in the extract above, this interviewee describes how persistent feelings of alienation eroded when hearing peers' experiences that mirror his own. Consequently, his self-categorisation as an inadequate person shifted to someone who had gained a sense of normalcy. Here, we see that the interviewee is particularly pleased that he could help others and was involved in a two-way process. In other words, he was able to adopt the role of '*supporter*' when aiding others.

In addition, groups offered hope and alternative explanations, which, in turn, limited the stigma attached to long-term unemployment, which is often accompanied by shame, guilt and self-recrimination. By gaining some perspective through reciprocity, interviewees could see the structural and shared underlying reasons behind individual experiences originating and existing outside themselves:

> This group has been really different to what I have at home. I live in a troubled family, and this is very different. This gives you a good kick, I think. It makes me think that there are other things in life, not just

what I have at home. Here, you encounter different people and you realise that other people aren't doing that well either. This provides some sort of new beginning to something, especially for those of us with long unemployment histories. Through this group, I can get some kind of ventilation to my brain. So, I am not only thinking about if I can afford to buy food. At least I have something to say to others.

(Client interview 10)

As seen here, being able to witness how others cope helps many clients shift their perspectives and self-reflect by recognising one another. In the extract above, the interviewee explains how she does not categorise herself and her situation as particularly 'problematic' based on the reciprocator role she adopted after sharing her experiences within the group setting.

Reciprocal acts may indeed provide a mechanism for redefining one's identity, maintaining a positive self-image and regaining control over one's life. This suggests that reciprocity plays a role in discrediting definitions of one's self (Hutchinson and Lovell 2013). Thus, the support group can affirm one's personal worth and individuality when one reflects on their own situation. In this way, one can recognise and understand shared experiences and co-construct them as well as self-categorise and reorient oneself in alternative ways. Reciprocity is particularly meaningful for those who depend upon others and are often conceptualised in a one-dimensional manner: as takers, passive recipients and 'burdens' to others (see Thompson 2013). In these terms, reciprocity is an important aspect of managing one's identity in relation to others because, without reciprocal encounters, one must manage an identity at the margins and in solitude.

Equally encountered

Clients described their previous relationships with service providers as typically unequal, asymmetrical and contractual. The vast majority of clients had previously experienced negative and humiliating encounters in welfare services; thus, the support group run by empathetic professionals became particularly helpful for many. Due to previous unpleasant experiences, clients stressed the importance of being at the 'same level' and being able to self-categorise themselves as equally encountered, as illustrated in the following:

We as a group have been quite talkative, and the professionals also share their thoughts and experiences. At first, I used a few swear words with my wife regarding why on earth I was put into this group. But, it was only because I didn't know what this was all about. I have enjoyed this group a lot. And, I really like the fact that professionals themselves participate in it. It is not like the normal interview situation.

(Client interview 12)

This interviewee categorises himself as occupying the same level as the professionals. This professional involvement challenged his previous experiences in professional-client relationships, in which he often felt that encounters represented a special hierarchical relationship, and he was simply an object of work in which the categorical difference was constructed in one way or another. In these relationships, professionals assume the roles of non-participating interviewers.

In general, according to clients, support groups offered an atmosphere filled with respect and recognition of them as fellow human beings. In addition, such groups facilitated authentic and trusting relationships characterised by blurred professional roles:

> We have had lots of humour and we've been able to speak about things using real terms; I think I got some hope through this group. I've really enjoyed the good sense of humour among professionals. All of us are on the same level, and most importantly they [professionals] do not look down on us – like uh 'we are professionals and we know'.
>
> (Client interview 13)

Clients emphasised the importance of not being looked down upon by professionals in these support group settings. Therefore, in contrast to controlling and bureaucratic encounters with professionals, feeling respected and on equal footing represented a particularly important experience for clients. Rosemary Green *et al.* (2006) believe that the expert and 'knower' role of social work professionals can create unnecessary boundaries, an imbalanced distribution of power and an artificial distance between the client and worker. Thus, I found that the support group experience broke down barriers between professionals and clients and, to a certain extent, challenged the power dynamics between them. As such, the dichotomy between professional and non-professional can be reconstructed and re-examined in order to achieve equity and reciprocity within social work practices.

Revised professional self-categorisation

In the following section, I focus on professionals' revised self-categorisations, which I identified in my analysis as *professionally grown* and *bystander*.

Professionally grown

The support group was not simply a one-way process. Professionals also reported benefitting from the experience. In general, the support group offered them a chance to critically re-examine their own practices and professional standings. However, this required some reflection and work by the professionals:

Through this group, I understand that the things that are good for me are not necessarily good for clients. So, if the client is satisfied – let's say by having booze – I can disagree with the client, but not look at him or her from a top-down perspective like unemployed clients are usually looked at. I have worked quite hard on this, or realised through this group that for many people to even come to a group like this and participate is a major effort.

(Professional interview 4)

In the extract above, the interviewee explains how the group experience allowed her to rethink her own attitudes and prejudices regarding the clients' ways of life, capabilities and service needs. This process also led to a critical reflection of the imbalance of power in the client-professional dynamic. Consequently, the interviewee sees herself as experiencing '*professional growth*' as a result of support group attendance.

Many professionals pointed out how they made a special effort to help clients feel appreciated and valued by avoiding judgemental views or by not 'stepping above' them. I understand this as a process of reciprocity and shared learning. Here, I agree with Sue Thompson (2016), who suggests promoting reciprocity and appreciating that feeling valued plays a key role in social work. This results from a value base espousing self-worth and importance because the core idea of the profession is to challenge a variety of discriminatory assumptions and practices.

Understanding how support groups helped professionals gain new roles also allows us to understand professional growth. The support group not only influenced the ways that professionals were perceived within the group but also how they were perceived outside the group in their daily practices:

I think this group provided a new situation for all of us, where both professionals and clients were in a group and talked together. I had some kind of a dual role. I normally work at a bureaucratic office, which is the only place where my clients meet me. So, now, due to this group, I noticed that clients perceive me and my working role at the office differently. It's easier for them to open up and share their thoughts at the office now when we've gone through this group together. In a way, this group changed my role at work quite a bit after I gave something of myself.

(Professional interview 1)

Here, the interviewee explains how the support group helped her clients see her beyond the bureaucratic role in her daily practice. As she explained, the successful support group experience required professionals to both give and receive. Interviewees explained how they shared their own experiences from their everyday lives, such as their struggles and difficulties around dieting, exercise and everyday activities. By giving something of themselves to the clients, professionals also reported gaining something in return, as we see in the extract above.

Carla Alexander and Grant Charles (2009) argue that a lack of reciprocity in welfare services may dehumanise and create artificial and restrictive barriers between clients and professionals. As we see above, the dual role of professionals is described as only positive; however, it may bring some complexities and challenges, both to clients and professionals. For example, exploitation and potential harm and damage to the client or professional may occur if such practices are not conducted ethically (see, for example, Reamer 2003, Pugh 2007).

Bystander

In addition, all of the professionals interviewed described various client-to-client support processes that helped clients validate and reaffirm themselves as valued citizens and contributors to society. This required an unusual role and level of activity from the professionals:

> I was really surprised how the clients started to share their thoughts openly and honestly, and how they gained trust between each other. We laughed and cried, and some clients had quite difficult stories to share. I was quiet quite a lot since the clients were supporting each other by giving each other tips and so on. It surprised me how human we were to one another. The clients first thought that the group was a sanction and coercive, but then it was something else. I was surprised – the same way they were.
>
> (Professional interview 1)

Here, the interviewee categorises herself as a *'bystander'* in the support group and its various helping processes. By not assuming a dominant role, clients had the opportunity to share their knowledge, skills, emotional support and experiences as reciprocators. Often, in welfare services, clients are described as being *in need* of help whilst simultaneously unable to *give* help and contribute to the well-being of others.

Professionals recognised the need to identify service-users' competencies to reciprocate at an organisational level. That is, support groups were viewed as a way of facilitating reciprocity and sharing.

> I was sort of withdrawing when clients started to speak about their shared experiences, like sleeping problems. They were sharing things that they found helpful and by sharing they were giving support to each other. It was somehow shocking to me that the clients did not previously have a place to share their experiences and deal with their life in its entirety. So, it feels to me that there is a real need for sharing experiences in this society.
>
> (Professional interview 4)

Here, the interviewee describes her '*bystander*' role as important to the support group's success. Professionals felt a real need for sharing and voicing their experiences among long-term unemployed individuals. Allowing for such experiences within welfare services is key because one's dignity may be affronted if insufficient opportunities exist for people to do things with and for other people (Thompson 2013, p. 7).

Conclusions

My analysis reflects the idea that in support groups, clients are identified beyond the compelling categories professionals and welfare institution providers use. Support groups offer not only a chance to be seen beyond specific categories but also the opportunity to assume new identities. This, in turn, simultaneously diminishes the self-blame and guilt felt by clients and enables professional growth amongst providers.

These results demonstrate that being recognised and treated as a valued human being beyond such categories represents vital experiences for those with prolonged unemployment histories. Therefore, individuals working within the social work profession should not view their clients as simply representing a harmful diagnosis or as problem cases. In particular, long-term unemployed social work clients may benefit from services that create a sense of normalcy and connectedness. This may also help clients to adopt a critical stance towards loaded and contested institutional and cultural categories rather than being confined by them.

We all rely on judgements from others, which provide additional opportunities for us to adapt and maintain positive self-images. These also allow for the formation of a positive identity, thus reshaping the stigmatised role of 'passive recipient' often assigned to unemployed individuals. From a social work perspective, how social work clients are viewed, how they see themselves and what kinds of labels are assigned to them remain crucial. Rather than relying on professional expertise related to the problem of unemployment, a greater range of critical voices should be heard regarding unemployment and its causes. These voices could be co-created through client-professional relationships as well as between peers. Relinquishing hierarchical relationships encourages positive client self-categorisations to emerge. It also confronts oppressive power dynamics, restrictive barriers and any separation between professionals and their clients, helping professionals to view themselves in new roles.

In addition, social work requires an understanding of the two-sided relationship and participation in reciprocal identity-making created through categorisation. Clients are not simply passive recipients of help and support; rather, they should be supported as active partners in various support processes. Therefore, social work as a field may move from imposing categories on clients to mutually enabling self-categorisation utilising various relationship-based practices to invoke alternative and positive categorisations constructed reciprocally (Juhila and Abrams 2011). In particular, social work that pursues change is based on a client's recourse, strengths and capacities, which, in turn, create positive identities (Juhila *et al.* 2014, p. 23). In social work among unemployed clients with complex histories and needs, greater effort could be directed towards addressing gradual and reciprocal processes and linking (as opposed to distancing) services not necessarily aimed at employment alone.

References

Alexander, C., and Charles, G., 2009. Caring, Mutuality and Reciprocity in Social Worker-Client Relationships. Rethinking Principles of Practice. *Journal of Social Work*, 9 (1), 5–22.

Caswell, D., Eskelinen, L., and Olesen, P., 2011. Identity Work and Client Resistance Underneath the Canopy of Active Employment Policy. *Qualitative Social Work*, 1 (1), 1–16.

Fook, J., 2002. *Social Work. Critical Theory and Practice.* London: SAGE Publications.

Green, R., Gregory, R., and Mason, R., 2006. Professional Distance and Social Work: Stretching the Elastic? *Australian Social Work*, 59 (4), 449–461.

Hjörne, E., Juhila, K., and van Nijnatten, C., 2010. Negotiating Dilemmas in the Practices of Street-level Welfare Work. *International Journal of Social Welfare*, 19 (3), 303–309.

Hutchinson, A., and Lovell, A., 2013. Participatory Action Research: Moving Beyond the Mental Health 'Service User' Identity. *Journal of Psychiatric Mental Health Nursing*, 20 (7), 641–649.

Juhila, K., and Abrams, L., 2011. Special Issue Editorial: Constructing Identities in Social Work Settings. *Qualitative Social Work*, 10 (3), 277–292.

Juhila, K., Günther, K., and Raitakari, S., 2014. Negotiating Mental Health Rehabilitation Plans: Joint Future Talk and Clashing Time Talk in Professional Client Interaction. *Time & Society*, 24 (1), 5–26.

Juhila, K., Pösö, T., Hall, C., and Parton, N., 2003. Introduction: Beyond a Universal Client. In Christopher Hall, Kirsi Juhila, Nigel Parton, and Tarja Pösö (eds.) *Constructing Clienthood in Social Work and Human Services. Interaction, Identities and Practices.* London: Jessica Kingsley Publishers, 11–26.

Karjalainen, V., 2014. Poliittisen harkinnan paradoksit. Kohderyhmänä pitkäaikaistyöttömät. In Laura Kalliomaa-Puha, Toomas Kotkas, and Marketta Rajavaara (eds.) *Harkittua? Avauksia sosiaaliturvan harkintavallan tutkimukseen.* Helsinki: Kelan tutkimusosasto, 114–133.

Keskitalo, E., 2008. Balancing Social Citizenship and New Paternalism Finnish Activation Policy and Street-level Practice in a Comparative Perspective. Helsinki: Stakes.

Kjørstad, M., 2016. Do Your Duty – Demand Your Right: A Theoretical Discussion of the Norm of Reciprocity in Social Work. *European Journal of Social Work*, doi:10.1080/13691457.2016.1246416.

Krogstrup, H., 1997. User Participation in Quality Assessment. A Dialogue and Learning Oriented Evaluation Method. *Evaluation*, 3 (2), 205–224.

Kroll, C., and Blomberg, H., 2011. Social Work-fare? Social workers' Views on the Poor, the Unemployed and Workfare-related Measures in Finland. In

H. Blomberg, and N. Kildal (eds.) *Workfare and Welfare State Legitimacy.* Helsinki: University of Helsinki, Nordic Centre of Excellence NordWel, 96–124.

Larsen, C., 2006. *The Institutional Logic of Welfare Attitudes. How Welfare Regimes Influence Public Support.* Ashgate: Hampshire.

Mäkitalo, Å., and Säljö, R., 2002a. Talk in Institutional Context and Institutional Context in Talk: Categories as Situated Practices. *Interdisciplinary Journal for the Study of Discourse*, 22 (1), 57–82.

Mäkitalo, Å., and Säljö, R., 2002b. Invisible People: Institutional Reasoning and Reflexivity in the Production of Services and "Social Facts" in Public Employment Agencies. *Mind, Culture, and Activity*, 9 (3), 160–178.

Närhi, K., and Kokkonen, T., 2014. Transformation of Participation Politics and Social Citizenship in Finnish Welfare Governance. In Aila-Leena Matthies, and Lars Uggerhoej (eds.) *Participation, Marginalisation and Welfare Services – Concepts, Politics and Practices Across European Countries.* Ashgate: Surrey, 95–112.

Pugh, R., 2007. Dual Relationships: Personal and Professional Boundaries in Rural Social Work. *British Journal of Social Work*, 37 (8), 1405–1423.

Reamer, F., 2003. Boundary Issues in Social Work: Managing Dual Relationships. *Social Work*, 48 (1), 121–133.

Roivainen, I., 2009. Does Community Work in Finland Benefit Citizens or Clients? In Gunn Strand Hutchinson (eds.) *Community Work in the Nordic Countries. New Trends.* Oslo: Universitetsforlaget, 98–118.

Tarkiainen, L., 2017. Long-term Unemployed Finnish Interviewees Address Deservingness: Separating, Declining and Enriching as Means of Resisting. *Journal of Poverty and Social Justice*, 25 (3), 219–231.

Thompson, S., 2013. *Reciprocity and Dependency in Old Age. Indian and UK Perspectives.* New York: Springer.

Thompson, S., 2016. Promoting Reciprocity in Old Age: A Social Work Challenge. *Social Work in Action*, 28 (5), 341–355.

6 Risk and reciprocity in residential care

Some problems with a universal norm

Claire Cameron

Introduction

Reciprocity is fundamental to well-being but is problematic in professional, hierarchical and intergenerational institutional care for children. But is this assertion just applicable to England? Might other social and cultural contexts offer alternative perspectives and methods of relationships in residential care?

Residential care is a place-based, institutional site for the care and supervision of young people, with the potential for other purposes, such as therapy or education. In contemporary England, and indeed Europe, residential care is diverse but most often characterised as a workplace for adults, usually organised into teams and working shift patterns, and a 'home' for young people, who live there, albeit often on a temporary basis, and whose 'basic' and 'safety' needs (Maslow 1943) should at least be met. Residential care in England can trace its roots to stigmatised care for impoverished children and families, and to housing young offenders (Berridge *et al.* 2011). By the early 1990s, it was regarded as a 'second best option staffed by a largely unqualified workforce' (*ibid.*, p. 4). Residential care offers care and supervision of young people, largely aged 12 and over, who have more serious difficulties, who have often been abused and neglected, and for whom family-based foster care has often failed. Residential care is for children with disabilities, usually as short breaks, or as secure accommodation, for young people whose own behaviour puts them at serious risk and as semi-independent accommodation for young people in the process of leaving care. There are also residential schools and therapeutic communities that offer more specialised support. In some cases, staff and their families live on-site. In total, over the year 2014–2015, 16, 340 young people in England lived in residential children's homes, secure units, residential schools or other residential settings (DfE 2015), representing 16.5 percent of all 'looked after' young people.

In other European countries, residential care is situated within an educative, or social pedagogic, framework and plays a proportionately bigger role as an option for children and young people in state care. For example, in Spain, Denmark and Germany, around half of all placements are in a residential institutional environment (Losada-Gistau *et al.* 2015, Ainsworth and Thoburn 2014).

Regardless of the rate of residential care use and the stated purpose – whether temporary refuge, longer term upbringing or reparative therapy – there is a common concern for the safety and well-being of children and young people. The milieu in which such concern is expressed is to a large extent through the relationships that are forged within the daily lives of the institutions. As Henry Maier (2016, p. 3) notes, residential care workers provide, for young people, 'the essential experience of being cared for, of learning how to respond and to interact'. Because children learn most from their immediate environments, workers hold pivotal positions and are 'always in the business of building a relationship, setting norms, and maintaining a linkage with society' (Maier und, p. 4). Workers are required to make fine-grained, in-the-moment judgements about practice at any given time; they are a presence, 'being there', focussed on the here and now and, in doing so, facilitating and/or joining in with young people's activities, depending on their assessments about what will work in any particular set of circumstances (Smith 2009). Residential care workers are, in fact, 'experts in everyday life' (Cameron *et al.* 2015). But is it possible for such an institution to be characterised by the social bonds of reciprocity?

Reciprocity is a universal norm around helping others and through which helping obligations are imposed (Gouldner 1960). As a concept, it rests on ideas of mutuality and temporally framed exchange. The act of being reciprocal can be considered through a framework of experience that changes over time and through culturally shaped norms and expectations. Reciprocity is the medium through which networks acquire meaning for social actors and so build social capital. Reciprocity has a self-interest and a social or community interest dimension to it: Actions are for the benefit of others and the social fabric of what is held in common as well as in the expectation of some return (Gauntlett unpub). Reciprocal action can be 'balanced', taking place among other people with similar needs, or 'generalised', which means that there is less or no expectation of return for largesse offered (Hansen 2005).

Reciprocity in the professional and 'home' environment of residential care might be expected to promote, reinforce and sustain the common purposes of care and education through the primary medium of relationships between adults and children, adults and adults, and the peer groups of young people. The professional role of residential care is situated within other networks, both professional- and community-oriented, that potentially offer reciprocal actions. Examples might be information exchange around young people and their needs and behaviours or give and take with neighbours to ensure amiable relations. One might expect to see relationships and activities within residential care homes that are characterised by mutual curiosity, joint learning and discovery, and kindness to the self and others. One might expect, in Axel Honneth's terms, to have recognition of one's own validity in the three dimensions of emotional, social and legal recognition (Honneth 1995).

However, residential care, perhaps particularly in England, also inhabits a contractual space, where the work is carried out according to plans that are specified and commissioned, in advance, for a placement fee. The professional exchanges that take place are accountable, not to the norm of reciprocity that is part of 'good citizenry' but to the contracted plans. The adult-child relationships are oriented, not through self- and altruistic or community interest in action and reward through re-action but to therapeutic and care purposes for individual young people. In this conceptualisation of residential care, relationships are largely hierarchical, where the workers offer, and young people receive. Furthermore, residential care workers are paid; their 'generalised' reciprocity may be better characterised as a helping professional (Smith and Smith 2008).

This chapter will examine some data from a study of social pedagogic approaches to child-adult relationships in residential care (Cameron 2013) to identify what scope for reciprocity there might be. One potential barrier for the operation of reciprocity is the influence of wider, societal discourses on practice in residential care. An example of such wider influences on practice examined here is risk. Risk is a dominant construction in child welfare work, certainly in the Anglo-American debate. James Anglin (2002) charts the rise of risk, and risk assessments, as part of a legalistic approach to child welfare, which has seen an increasing emphasis on the determination of possible future risk or an 'educated prediction' about what will happen. This is in line with Ulrich Beck's (1992) outline of a 'risk society' that is oriented towards a negative and defensive image of the future in which risk assessment is about preventing, or insulating against the effects of, perceived problems that may occur. Indeed, risk thinking curtails taking risks and encourages risk aversion among child welfare professionals (Anglin 2002). Arguably, it is part of the commissioned plans for children living in residential care and cuts across notions of reciprocity. If risk assessments involve experts from outside the residential care setting deciding what is and is not (too) risky for children to do, or professionals being alerted to possible risks from a particular activity via writing everything down in advance, does this compromise the essential character of reciprocal actions based on mutuality? Does risk thinking inhibit the building of relationships and networks that may offer both practical opportunities and social capital to young people? The second section of data in this chapter examines ways in which risk is conceptualised in residential care in a cross-national context. I will conclude by offering an alternative to reciprocity as a conceptual frame for residential care: an adaptation of recognition theory.

The study

The aim of the study was to investigate how relational practice was conceptualised from the perspective of professionals who were expert in the field of working with children and young people in Belgium, Denmark and

Germany. A comparative design was selected, with a view to contributing to the debate in England about how to improve relational practice and make residential placements more successful (Hetherington 2006). The countries were chosen to reflect differences in the organisation of, and cultural approaches to, practice with children as compared to England (Cameron 2013). All three belonged to what Neil Gilbert (1997) termed a 'family service' orientation to child welfare. By contrast, England's approach to child welfare is 'child protection', which treats family support and child protection as discrete systems and is more crisis-oriented (Hetherington 2006).

Data sources

Thirty-seven in-depth interviews were held (in 2011–12), with key stakeholders from policy (n=8), research (9), professional education (5), trade unions (5) and practice (10) in the three continental countries (13 in Denmark; 11 in Flanders; 13 in Germany). In addition, six similar interviews were carried out with social pedagogues who held a tertiary degree studies in Social Pedagogy from Germany and had worked in residential care in England.[1] The latter group were included to identify differences between social pedagogic knowledge and practice in other countries and that of their English colleagues.[2] Study participants were identified via opportunistic snowballing by a key contact in each country in as few administrative areas as possible. This was done to minimise any variations in policy implementation across areas. In Belgium, the focus of enquiry was Flanders, the largest of the country's autonomous regions, and, in Germany, fieldwork took place in Hessen and Baden Württemberg. In Denmark, fieldwork was carried out in Copenhagen and the immediate area around it. The interviews in England were geographically dispersed, depending on where the social pedagogues had been employed and had settled. The six participants had previously worked for three local authorities and two voluntary sector organisations. In total, there were four country-specific sets of data.

Method

Interview schedules included perceptions of the wider discourse around children and young people and those in the care of the state; concepts, theories and how they relate to practice; and practice and the organisation of practice. Interviews were recorded via contemporaneous note-taking and/or digital recorder, typed and returned to study participants for checking and amendment. Analysis proceeded by: i) compiling country-based reports, synthesising the data from each set of interviews and available national level documentation, and adding to already compiled background reports; ii) writing summaries for each country and circulating these to study participants; iii) thematic analysis guided by the main areas of the interview schedule; and iv) comparative analysis in a country context.

Reciprocity within four types of relationships

Study participants' responses to an open question about the purpose of child-professional relationships revealed four ways of conceptualising them:

Building skills

The child or young person is envisaged as a person whose social being requires additional skills in order to participate in society, and the professional, through advising, modelling and sharing lifespace in a non-judgemental way, can help the children gain confidence, strengthen their abilities, support their development and learn how to behave in the social world. Study participants from all four data sets referred to this purpose of relationships, which was categorised as 'a vehicle for the development of self and skills'.[3] Examples were given, such as a social pedagogue going to live with a father and son in a situation in which the father was psychotic, and the social authorities needed to identify whether or not the son could continue to live with the father. The pedagogue focussed on *doing things* with the father to build up a relationship that could withstand a potentially very difficult message. The study participant said

> The pedagogue sits together with them and is sad together with them. The decision is made in the professional team through a lot of discussion about what it means, what can we deal with, how much pressure can the father stand. The team supports one professional to work on the case.

In another example, five Danish social pedagogues worked with one 14-year-old in order to

> start from the beginning, teaching him how to get up in the morning, wash, place things in the room, he had a strange way of piling up things on the floor. And they took all the fights with him, but they were genuinely interested in him. Everything from the beginning – after approximately one year he begun to trust them. He could pick the one he trusted at a time. [They] did lots of interesting things together.

In both of these cases, study participants discussed a situation as a 'dilemma', rather than a problem, to be resolved. Arguably, 'dilemma' positions the situation on a more mutual footing than 'problem' does. Sharing the lifespace of a family's home or residential setting, with 'genuine interest', and 'doing things together' also emphasises mutuality and joint discovery, and provides opportunities to convey empathy as in 'we sit together' and are 'sad together'. Sharing the lifespace also enables predictable, and socially and culturally accepted, routines to be established, which are modelled by social pedagogues and learned by young people over time. The work of the pedagogue is done within a professional team, the members of which support, analyse and reflect upon the practice and its progress together. The aim is that increased well-being is achieved through action, and it creates the conditions for trust to be established between the parties, which, in turn, increases the confidence of the young person to act themselves.

Reciprocity might be visible in the detail of doing things together, but social pedagogues' professional responsibilities are about resolving dilemmas and modelling behaviour and learning. This is arguably much less reciprocal. Combined with team analysis and action, the pedagogue brings greater power, responsibility and authority to bear on the relationship.

An ethical encounter

In this approach, professionals' relationships with young people were without an ulterior purpose. Instead, relationships were seen as providing an opportunity to be supportive to a young person, to 'work at the notion of human dignity', to 'be there' for a young person, and to create an environment in which a young person perceived the adult to 'be special' to them. Here, the purpose of being in relation was about learning how to live together. One study participant, a manager from a children's home and family support service in Flanders, said, 'we are focused on settings, and creating places in which people can come to reflect and do things together. Find ways to engage. Even if there are problems with parents'. Another Flemish study participant argued that

> the relation is necessary, and perhaps the only thing you have to do is install that relation. As a starting point. The rest is to be defined within what is happening there. Of course what is the quality of care, what we think we will work or help or solve. The relation has no purpose, because purpose leads to an instrumental dimension.

This approach might be termed an *'ethical encounter'* because the 'here and now' has meaning, and the actions of professionals are designed to convey the message that 'you are worthwhile [and] just as I find you important, you mean something to me' (Flanders, psychologist). The point of the encounter is authentic connection with young people. A Flemish trade union representative said,

> it is important to follow these young people from a pedagogical perspective. A large number of professionals really connect with the children. They see what the children need – and this is frustrating to see what they need but to not be able to fill the responsibility you have. In general the young people and the professionals connect.

The idea of professionals and young people forming a 'connection' and 'being there' is arguably on a different level than meeting need or building skills, although there are similarities in terms of professional actions and environment. Even more than in the first 'purpose' discussed, mutual meaning-making is to the fore. There is a concern to eliminate, as far as possible, institutionalised hierarchies in which staff (adults) know best, and 'living together' is seen as a project to work on in itself. Arguably, there is more potential here for reciprocity to flourish because professionals see themselves as inhabiting the same level of expertise (more or less) as young people. For example, one study participant said that at times, it can be important to say, 'bugger off' to a young person as part of a working relationship to create an environment that allows young people to ask their own questions, talk about their own needs, and allows staff to ask young people what they think is important and say what is on offer.

A vehicle for emancipation

Professional-child relationships were seen as holding the potential to 'give voice' to children, who are positioned as less powerful than adults but for whom opportunities to express autonomy could be created. A practitioner from Flanders believed that the first principle of practice was 'to give the child a grip on his own life, so that he can develop and go further, with or without his parents ... [and that the practitioner should identify] what possibilities for action, give child a voice'. A trade union representative from Germany concurred that 'the professional gives the opportunity to have a voice. The key word is to give opportunities, to use opportunities; you have to create the good conditions'. Respondents in both Flanders and Germany referred to the importance of participation in the structures of society, including the services children attend (Milova 2008), as participation gives young people essential life skills for negotiation and making choices (Winkler 2000).

In this conceptualisation, mutual reciprocity is less important than 'giving' voice. Adults create the conditions in which young people can express themselves, make choices and exercise autonomy. Part of these conditions is affording young people legal and social recognition in societal structures, such as residential care services, so that they may participate meaningfully. Social recognition comes through 'giving' validity to the young people's viewpoints, which arguably has a more overtly political project. The language of 'giving' also suggests that the starting point is hierarchical, unequal positioning of adults-professionals, who have the power to 'give', and children-residents, who are recipients. Moreover, such inequality is relinquished at a pace decided by adults.

Gain a professional understanding of a child's problem

The most commonly cited conceptualisation was of relationship as an opportunity to gain the trust of the young person so that they were able to tell the professional about their difficulties. With this knowledge, a practitioner would be able to make changes in the young person's life and/or make their relationships with their birth parents bearable. For example, a practitioner from Germany thought the purpose was

> to get a change from before ... if there is no relationship, if they don't believe I have a good idea, it's difficult to get them to do something different, or even to tell them something about themselves ... the big issue is how can we speak together ... it's important he tells me so I can understand.

Practitioners should be very active and reliable; as one practitioner in Flanders said, 'very often the child is impressed by what we know – and that it's straight – that they can trust what I say is what I mean. It has to be open communication'. The purpose of the pedagogues' work with child is ensuring 'that the relationship with their own family is bearable. Or is improving'.

This type of relationship was also less concerned with reciprocity in terms of mutual exchange. Young people were seen as individuals who were in need of a confidante who could help them address their 'underlying issues', 'achieve change' and 'express their self differently'. This is a more therapeutically oriented relationship, in which the pedagogue has a duty to help resolve potentially painful emotional difficulties through the young person's releasing personal information about themselves. The goal is for pedagogues to be the person young people want to 'spend time' with, who can 'help with anything'. A dominant theme in this account is 'trust'. Rather than using the language of mutuality and co-construction, trust relies on taking a risk that one's choices will not be disappointed (Luhmann 2000). It is not the same as rational calculation of the risk of being disappointed because trust is only required if 'a bad outcome would make you regret your action' (Luhmann 2000, p. 98). In a residential setting, trust is the first of seven elements of caring relationships and is made up of reliability and confidentiality (Laursen 2003). In Erik Laursen's study, young people appeared to have a higher bar for trust than in the definition given by Niklas Luhmann in that they would only ascribe trust to practitioners who had already proven their trustworthiness. In the current study, practitioners largely concurred with Laursen's findings: Trust was a demonstrable alignment between verbal commitment and action. From this perspective, professionals have a responsibility to prove themselves trustworthy through their actions as the one in whom young people can invest their knowledge and feelings.

So far, the data suggests that two types of professional-child relationships within the framework of social pedagogy are oriented towards reciprocity (building skills, an ethical encounter), but two others (vehicle for emancipation, gaining a professional understanding) are not. Moreover, the latter two types were the most commonly found. Barriers to reciprocity are generational status inequalities between adults (practitioners) and children (residents), young people's practical and emotional need for help and support with everyday life, and differences in the representation of 'home' for young people and 'work' for practitioners (Clark *et al.* 2014).

Risk as a potential barrier to reciprocity

A further potential barrier to reciprocity in residential care settings is the discourse of risk, risk aversion and its accompanying sibling, fear of allegations. Study participants were asked how risk was thought about in their professional domains and specifically whether written risk assessments were used.[4] They were also asked about the role of physical touch in professional-child relationships. There were wide differences between the responses in the three continental European countries compared to the reported practice in England.

Discourse of risk in residential care in England

The impact of a discourse of risk on everyday life and work in residential care was said to be twofold: bureaucratic and pedagogic. Risk thinking involved considerable paperwork, which was a bureaucratic burden on staff and young people. Study participants said that in some cases, there were up to 42 'generic' risk assessments already prepared for different eventualities, such as 'going swimming, going on the moors'. One said that 'sometimes [young people] would ask for things like go to a leisure centre on the weekends, perfectly ordinary things, and they would have to wait while you filled in the paperwork'.

Second, the perception of risk shaped which activities were considered acceptable and which were best avoided. A study informant claimed that risk assessments were required for 'a walk in the park. To play board games! I had to sign a risk assessment for board games. I was shocked'. Assessing the risk of such ordinary everyday activities compromised the knowledge and skills of professionally trained social pedagogues. As one said, 'I know the risks whether they are written down or not'. Another reported that in her former employment in Germany, one was

> working in a professional setting [that is] is a dynamic risk assessment and you have to know when it is appropriate to say no – say bungee jumping. But if we wanted to go cycling and camping and there were agreements beforehand but it's not on paper [it was OK].

The perception of risk noted as a powerful influence on the pedagogy of everyday life, with consequences, the social pedagogues thought, on the broad development of self and skills.

Risk-taking as natural

One study participant had found that there was a 'risk aversion for things which children would normally explore in family, such as outdoor activities'. Social pedagogues thought it was 'natural' to climb a wall, but if a resident did it, 'everyone screams about the danger'. Another said that the prospect of a young person getting hurt 'makes it difficult to take risks. But accidents can happen. If we allow a cycle ride, it is a risk. It needs a better balance. The young people often miss out on exploring abilities'. She also said that 'making a fire whilst camping is often not [thought] possible. I did it once and it was safe'.

Missing out on learning

The theme of missing out on learning by avoiding risk recurred. For example, one study participant said,

> children need the right to let them make risky decisions. Let them hurt their leg and fall down. If we don't let them be afraid, when they live on their own they will be and it's not fair on them.

Failing to allow risks to be taken in everyday life did not help young people when they left residential care, the interviews claimed. Up until the age of 16,

> everything is done, they don't have to do anything; then overnight at age 16 everything changes. There is no contingency plan. What parents do for years, here is done in two weeks with the most traumatised children. And then everyone wonders why it doesn't work out.

Failure to protect

Some study participant social pedagogues contrasted risk aversion practices in the homes with what they perceived as a failure to protect residents. One said,

> we are not allowed to lock the doors at night. The young people can leave the house when they want. In Germany I had to visit their friends to make sure they were suitable. Here we don't know who they are with at all. We have no rights to do anything to keep them safe. We are not allowed to go into their room. I would make it harder for them to get out during the night.

A second concurred, 'we can't keep them in, we let them run out of the house, a 14 year old with history of sexual exploitation, we can report them as missing. But we can't lock them in'.

Fear of allegations

Practice was also shaped by a fear of allegations being made against practitioners. This was particularly reported in relation to the use of physical touch. All the social pedagogues referred to the importance of physical touch as a source of comfort and security for young people in residential care. In one example, a study participant said,

> the quality of touch is that it covers things that can't be expressed in words, if you ask for a hug, in a situation where there is conflict or grief, and there are no words to make the situation good. To give a hug or sit together close, is very helpful and important.

Another said,

> I was sitting at a computer typing away and a boy asked for a hug and I got up and hugged him tight. He was surprised and the staff were open mouthed. He did not think he would get a hug when he asked for it.

The social pedagogues also talked about the therapeutic potential of massage and the ways in which this was negotiated in their settings. One reported that

> In the beginning I said how is it with massage. I was not trained as such but I have some skills. They said it was not allowed. I asked where it was written down that it was not allowed. It wasn't. I said I would do it in the living room, with the doors open. I massaged the feet of a young girl while we were watching TV. She asked me to do it again. It had a good effect. We had a boy who was difficult, settling at bedtimes. He first observed me massaging, and then asked me if he could have a neck and shoulders massage. I asked him to shower and put on fresh clothes, which was often a matter for dispute. He watched TV while I massaged him. I could feel his tension in his shoulders releasing. ...
>
> With another boy we had a breakthrough using massage. I decided not to ask questions about it. Then colleagues were asked to massage the young people, and they did. There was no adverse reaction from staff. I said to the other staff about my conditions – that they should be fully clothed, doors open, public places. They could tell it had good effects, saw that the boy had a shower and went to bed which was not always the case. But it was not discussed in the round.

Another study participant reported that when a boy asked if she could give him a massage, she consulted a member of staff and agreed that

> if two of us were in the room and it was sitting down on a chair with clothes on [it would be OK]. She was there as a witness. There was a fear of allegations. I said to him no problem. After 30 minutes it was done. We talked about it at the end of the shift, and they all said I was putting myself at risk, because I was not a trained masseur and would get sued.

I would do that if my own child asked for it, it was on the shoulders and there was a witness and it was recorded.

These findings suggest that risk is considered, in the experience of these social pedagogues working in residential care in different parts of England, as a negative and defensive concept that aims at preventing something worse happening (Beck 1992). The social pedagogues, however, had a different perspective, much of which was based on physicality: Exploring how the body can manage the environment was seen as foundational for learning; feeling the contact with another human being through touch was seen as a source of comfort and security.

Discourse of risk in Denmark, Germany and Flanders

There was much less consensus across responses to the question of conceptualising risk in Denmark, Germany and Flanders, indicating that the debate was much less developed according to study participants in these countries than in England. The main themes were about the close association between learning and risk-taking, the situated judgement of practitioners in weighing up different options and possibilities for young people, accompanying young people when going to visit places and people outside the institution, and assessing risk as part of everyday life and work in residential care. In common with the social pedagogues in England, study participants in all three countries referred to the value of learning through experience, in which taking risks was inevitable.

A Danish study participant considered risk 'part of life, all our children get in trouble sometimes', and some 'don't feel they live unless they are hanging off a cliff'. German participants argued that the aim of practice was to expose children to as many learning opportunities as possible, individually and in groups, to enable them to acquire skills and knowledge that would help them to adapt to life in society when they left care. Resistance of a risk discourse, in which 'we have to prevent all kinds of risks', was prevalent among some study participants in Flanders, who believed that 'physical risks are seen as part of learning'.

While German study participants agreed that, as one said, 'our job' ... [is to] 'to protect them from harm', precise and excessive regulation of risk was seen as impossible and stifling. Rules about recording young people's whereabouts and ensuring their safety during activities exist, but where there are situations of risk, practitioners have to use their professional judgment.

Study participants referred to responding to risk situations in terms of 'practice dilemmas' that require debate. The dilemma of, for example, 'when we know that this young girl communicates on the internet to meet a man – but we can't deny her to go to town' is an opportunity to debate the tension between safety and giving sufficient freedom so that young people can have experiences that are similar to those of other young people their age.

One study participant from Flanders concluded,

> Sometimes we prevent children from having experiences. Sometimes it doesn't work out well, this is life. We learn by experience. If you know that experience will be detrimental, it's better not to, for example, try cocaine, some groups are very vulnerable to develop addictions. But it's ... a difficult job, you have to take the decisions, and sometimes you have to make the right decision to let them go out and you may only know afterwards that it's the right decision.

Beyond the value of risk as an opportunity for learning, responses to the question of risk were diverse and referred to, for example, the risk of accidents and professional burnout; birth parents' concerns about the risk behaviours of young people; risk that birth parents might represent to young people; risk of violence or bullying in residential care groups; and risk associated with legal responsibilities, such as giving out medicines or driving an institution's van. One German study participant summed up the general bemusement at the question by saying that the concept that the carer might create risk for the young person does not exist as 'social pedagogues and social workers still have the image of themselves as 'carers' and don't put children at risk'. In striking contrast to the experience of practice in England, no study participants referred to written risk assessments. When prompted, responses were that such a procedure was 'very bureaucratic. We don't have that. Written risk assessments are not known'.

Risk and reciprocity

The discourse on risk in child welfare work is clearly very different in England to that in Flanders, Denmark and Germany. The unanimity of the responses in England, compared to the diversity elsewhere, suggests a pervasive risk discourse that had a deep impact on everyday practice and life in children's homes. The most immediate impact on reciprocity is that risk thinking and particularly written risk assessments predominated. Risk thinking had its origins in the wider societal and bureaucratic context and effectively shaped the adult-professional and young person-resident relationships and activities. This cuts across reciprocity and obliges professionals to carry out procedures, regardless of their professional judgement. For instance, cycling was procedurally regarded as a risk activity. Promoting cycling is government policy (Department of Transport 2015), but for children in residential care, it requires a risk assessment. Apart from the prospect of young people being denied their rights to enjoy leisure time, the involvement of a third party (externally imposed risk assessments) obstructs the educative potential of engaging young people in relational dialogue about 'risky' or dangerous activity. Diverting responsibility for initiating the definition and assessment of risk to an external body can represent lost opportunities for staff and young people to make decisions together or to practice the kind of decision-making young people will go through when they are independent adults. 'Missing out on learning' is also missing out on opportunities for reciprocal, educative mutual curiosity about what a young person wants to do, where they want to go, who they want to be with, what they might face there and so on. In contrast, the responses in the continental European countries was of rules made at the local – institutional – level to ensure safety and of *accompanying* young people. This indicates a localised, relationally led decision-making about what is good, and safe, for young people, with more potential for reciprocal action.

Conclusion

The social pedagogic relationships studied fell into four broad types. Only two of these, named here as 'building skills' and 'an ethical encounter', could be described as promoting reciprocity. The others were more instrumental and saw the relationship as a means to acquire children's trust, and their information, and to give them a voice in their own lives. While all four types rely on the expertise and professional responsibility of the adult, the latter two emphasise the hierarchical inequality of the adult-child relationship to a greater extent, which arguably mitigates reciprocity. Clearly, not all aspects of the professional role and the extent to which they may or may not act reciprocally are represented in the data presented here. For example, there is scant attention to residential care practitioners role within professional networks or with birth parents. But the mutuality dimension of reciprocity is given expression within the general social pedagogic ideas of 'sharing lifespace', 'doing things together' and practice as 'dilemmas' rather than problems. This possibility for reciprocity was thrown into sharp relief when the findings on risk were discussed. Risk is a far more dominant discourse in the accounts of practice in England compared with those from the other three countries. The apparatus of risk, risk assessment and risk management had a clear impact on everyday activities, from delaying the timing of activities to subjecting them to thorough scrutiny or prohibiting them altogether. As constituted in the accounts of social pedagogues working in England, risk thinking was a barrier to reciprocal activities in relationships as it required the practitioners to carry out externally prescribed rules and procedures rather than assessing the likelihood of danger in the moment and in the context of the relationship, the individuals and their capabilities, and the learning that could be gained from taking risks.

It would appear that the 'universal norm' of reciprocity is subject to serious constraint in (English) residential care. Once translated into the professional, hierarchical and regulated institutional environment, reciprocity has a marginal place, although there are examples of residential communities that work at challenging these ideas and promoting mutuality and respect, such as therapeutically oriented Camphill-Steiner (Jackson 2011) and drug treatment collectives in Norway (Lone 2010).

Perhaps a stronger conceptual framework is offered by developing Honneth's theory of recognition, as adapted by Hanne Warming (2015) and Nigel Thomas *et al.* (2016). For these authors, emotional recognition is the idea that one must not only receive love and care but also give it, throughout all life phases, not just in early childhood. This approach validates relations in residential care that include warmth and affection; gives a rationale for physical touch, such as a hug; and provides a context for massage as a helpful form of physical contact. Legal recognition includes being regarded as morally responsible and sharing citizen rights, regardless of whether a child lives in a family or a residential home, and being supported in doing so. In this reading, residential care workers would have an obligation to support children's rights to participation, and reliance on externally imposed procedures to control risk would be superseded by institutional and practice-level responsibilities to assess participation in the context of what is possible and its potential benefits. Finally, social recognition opens the way for young people's talents and strengths to be valued in the communities in which they live. Adoption of participation-oriented recognition in residential care would move away from a focus on the adult-child dichotomy that consideration of reciprocity leads to while still allowing for the mutuality, learning and warmth of relationships that are the foundation of good care and education.

Acknowledgements

This research was financially supported by Anglia Ruskin University. Dr Roxana Anghel, Anglia Ruskin University, assisted with data collection and analysis. Professor Michel Vandenbroeck, University of Ghent; professor Andreas Walther, University of Frankfurt; and Inge Danielsen, University College Copenhagen, assisted with access to study participants. I am grateful to all, including study participants.

Notes

1 Ethical permission was granted by Anglia Ruskin University Ethics Committee.
2 Social pedagogues (or their variants) are the major occupational role working with young people in care and education settings in many European countries and further afield (Cameron and Moss 2011).
3 All indented excerpts are from transcribed data.
4 Written risk assessments are a part of the everyday working environment in children's homes in England.

References

Ainsworth, F. and Thoburn, J., 2014. An Exploration of the Differential Usage of Residential Childcare Across National Boundaries. *International Journal of Social Welfare*, 23 (1), 16–24.

Anglin, J., 2002. Risk, Well-Being, and Paramountcy in Child Protection: The Need for Transformation. *Child and Youth Care Forum*, 31 (4), 233–255.

Beck, U., 1992. *Risk Society: Towards a New Modernity.* London: Sage.

Berridge, D., Biehal, N. and Henry, L., 2011. *Living in Children's Residential Homes.* Department for Education Research Report 2011.

Cameron, C., 2013. Cross-National Understandings of the Purpose of Professional-Child Relationships: Towards a Social Pedagogical Approach. *International Journal of Social Pedagogy*, 2 (1), 3–16.

Cameron, C. and Moss, P. ed., 2011. *Social Pedagogy and Working with Children and Young People: Where Care and Education Meet.* London: Jessica Kingsley.

Cameron, C., Reimer, D. and Smith, M., 2015. Towards a Theory of Upbringing in Foster Care in Europe. *European Journal of Social Work*, doi: 10.1080/13691457. 2015.1030360.

Clark, A., Cameron, C. and Kleipoedszus, S., 2014. Sense of Place in Children's Residential Care Homes: Perceptions of Home? *Scottish Journal of Residential Child Care*, 13 (2), 1–18.

Department for Education, 2015. Children looked after in England (including adoption and care leavers) year ending 31 March 2015, SFR 34, available from: https://www.gov.uk/government/uploads/system/uploads/attachment_data/file/464756/SFR34_2015_Text.pdf [accessed 15 August 2016].

Department of Transport, 2015. Local Transport. Available from: https://www.gov.uk/government/policies/local-transport [accessed 15 August 2016].

Gauntlett, D., und. *Three Approaches to Social Capital.* Available from www.makingisconnecting.org [accessed 15 August 2016].

Gilbert, N. ed., 1997. *Combatting Child Abuse: International Perspectives and Trends.* New York/Oxford: Oxford University Press.

Gouldner, A., 1960. The Norm of Reciprocity: A Preliminary Statement. *American Sociological Review*, 25 (2), 161–178.

Hansen, K., 2005. *Not-so-nuclear Families: Class, Gender and Networks of Care.* New Brunswick: Rutgers University Press.

Hetherington, R., 2006. Learning from Difference: Comparing Child Welfare Systems. In: N. Freymond and G. Cameron, eds. *Towards Positive Systems of Child and Family Welfare.* University of Toronto Press: Toronto, 27–50.

Honneth, A., 1995. *The Struggle for Recognition: The Moral Grammar of Social Conflicts.* Cambridge: Polity Press.

Jackson, R., ed. 2011. *Discovering Camphill: New Perspectives, Research and Developments.* Edinburgh: Floris Books.

Laursen, E. K., 2003. Seven Habits of Reclaiming Relationships. *Reclaiming Children and Youth*, 11 (1), 10–14.

Lone, A., 2010. Collectives – a Norwegian Success Story in Residential Care for Drug Addicts Based on a Social Pedagogical Approach. *European Journal of Social Education*, 18–19, 60–72.

Losada-Gistau, J., Montserrat, C. and Casas, F., 2015. The Subjective Well-being of Adolescents in Residential Care Compared to that of the General Population. *Children and Youth Services Review*, 52, 150–157.

Luhmann, N., 2000. Familiarity, Confidence, Trust: Problems and Alternatives. In: D. Gambetta ed. *Trust: Making and Breaking Cooperative Relations.* Available from: http://www.nuffield.ox.ac.uk/users/gambetta/Trust_making%20and%20breaking%20cooperative%20relations.pdf [accessed 15 August 2016].

Maier, H., und. *Children and Youth Grow and Develop in Group Care.* Available from: http://www.cyc-net.org/CYR101C/pdf/maier-develop.pdf [accessed 15 August 2016].

Maslow, A., 1943. A Theory of Human Motivation. *Psychological Review*, 50, 370–396.

Milova, H., 2008. *Participation of Children and Young People Living in Institutional Care.* Outcome Network Issue 3. Available from: http://www.outcome-network.org/paper/167:participation_of_children_and_young_people_living_in_institutional_care [accessed 15 August 2016].

Smith, H. and Smith, M. K., 2008. *The Art of Helping Others. Being Around, Being There, Being Wise.* London: Jessica Kingsley.

Smith, M., 2009. *Rethinking Residential Child Care.* Bristol: Policy Press.

Thomas, N., Graham, A., Powell, M. and Fitzgerald, R., 2016. Conceptualisations of Children's Well-being at School: The Contribution of Recognition Theory. *Childhood*, 1–15, doi: 10.1177/0907568215622802.

Warming, H., 2015. The Life of Children in Care in Denmark: A Struggle Over Recognition. *Childhood*, 22 (2), 248–262.

Winkler, M., 2000. Diesseits der Macht. Partizipation *In*: "Hilfen zur Erziehung" – Annäherungen an ein komplexes Problem, Neue Sammlung. Vierteljahres-Zeitschrift für Erziehung und Wissenschaft.1, 189–209.

7 Reciprocity and relationship-based approach in child welfare

Riitta Vornanen and Pirjo Pölkki

Introduction

The importance of reciprocal relationships was on the agenda in the early discussions of social work scholars. Mary Richmond delivered a paper at a conference in 1901, highlighting the family as an entity and a dynamic interpersonal process, and stressing the social context in which individuals seek belonging and meaning (Wood 2001, p. 18). Richmond's colleague Porter Lee examined the family as a system with reciprocal relationships in 1919 (Wood 2001, p. 18). The topic of reciprocal relationships is not new to social work, but it needs revisiting in light of current debate and research. For example, among the questions raised in Finland and elsewhere in the 1990s, after ratification of the Convention on the Rights of the Child, was whether children are visible and heard, and able to participate in welfare systems (Pölkki 1992). Debate continues on the dynamics of vulnerable children's invisibility, although it is now more in connection with communication and psychosocial work with this group (Ferguson 2016b). The concept of reciprocity prompts consideration of the crucial role of relationships in child welfare: How are the needs of children and families understood and met?

Child welfare work intervenes in relationships, regardless of the child policy or context of the work. Our interest centres on how Finnish child welfare has developed under the Nordic welfare state model, wherein social welfare is organised locally in municipalities. Finland's child welfare has been built on a philosophy whereby public authorities have a right to intervene in families (Hearn et al. 2004). Child welfare social workers have been responsible for leading child welfare processes, but the intensive work with families has often been the duty of family workers guided by social workers (Pölkki et al. 2016). In international comparison, Finland's child welfare system has been described as both family service-oriented and child-focussed rather than focussed narrowly on child protection (Gilbert 1997, Gilbert et al. 2011, Pösö 2011). The tradition of child welfare was built in the context of bureaucratic municipal social welfare, and Finland faces the challenge of developing routes to more intensive work with families in child welfare (STM 2013). Developments in Finland have inspired our efforts and discussions around the possibilities of relationship-based approaches to child welfare, with special focus on elements of reciprocal relationships and their significance in supporting relationships within child welfare social work. The relationship-based approach is not new in clinical work and is the subject of in-depth international research (e.g. Ruch and Julkunen 2016). However, we argue that the concept of reciprocity is not widely discussed in child welfare research in Finland or internationally.

The goal of child welfare is to sustain and support a safe environment for the child's growth. The requirement and ultimate aim is to guarantee safe, reciprocal relationships and a sense of belonging within a family or in out-of-home care. Finnish child policy is aimed at supporting families in their child-rearing duties by means of family policy, allowances and services. Private family life is protected by the European Convention on Human Rights (Article 8). Family relations are in the realm of private family life, and interventions are carefully regulated via codes of professional ethics and the law.

The current model of Finnish child welfare is built on the principle of gradually strengthening interventions and support. Its first level is preventive: supporting families via family policy and basic services, such as schooling and early education (Pölkki and Vornanen 2016). The idea is for society to support all families in taking care of their children and in the development of reciprocal relationships. The second level is support via family services in accordance with the Social Welfare Act (2014/1301), which allows social workers to provide support and services in line with assessments of service needs. The third level constitutes responses to a child at risk or in need of child welfare support or child protection measures (Child Welfare Act 2007/417). When considering private family life and reciprocal relationships in a family, it can be assumed that there are ethically charged and sensitive issues involved, with even higher levels of tension in situations concerning families with child welfare problems. Relationships within the family may affect relationships with professionals and how help is sought and received (Gladstone *et al.* 2014, p. 56).

When intervening in the life of a family, child welfare intervenes in intimate relationships, and a social worker becomes a part of the system. The boundaries of the social work relationship are negotiated and reflected from the perspective of reciprocity (O'Leary *et al.* 2013). The efforts of child welfare social workers are aimed at supporting direct relationships between a child and his/her parents as well as direct relationships with the child. A heavy caseload, bureaucratic demands or missing opportunities to direct relationship-based work may cause disappointment and intervention in family life without positive outcomes for the child and the family (Winter *et al.* 2017). This has also been a challenge in Finland, where caseloads have been heavy, and work has been done under the pressure of bureaucratic and required legal duties. There are also worker- and context-related issues that influence how reciprocity is constructed in child welfare.

The more a family is involved with various professionals, the more its internal relationships and complicated dynamics may be revealed in professional assessments. This chapter focusses on reciprocity and the relationship-based approach and discusses relations between children and parents, parents and social workers, and children and social workers. Based on selected interdisciplinary studies, we analyse enabling mechanisms and barriers to reciprocal relationship-based and reflective work with children and families. We also discuss and give some examples of ways of supporting reciprocal relationships and security among vulnerable clients.

Reciprocity and relationship-based approaches in the context of child welfare

The concept of reciprocity refers to the positive aspects of being in contact with another person and being capable of responding to others' needs. It is an essential phenomenon in social relations and social exchange. Variations in the structure of reciprocity influence the bonds of trust (Molm 2010, p. 119). In this pattern of mutual exchange, people are supposed to get something and give something back. The word has many positive connotations and explanations (in connection with social capital, see Diekmann 2004, p. 489). According to Linda D. Molm (2010, p. 120), reciprocity is a process that varies with the form of exchange. It has profound consequences for social relationships. It involves the use of power and also the emergence of trust and solidarity. Reciprocity is visible in its most elementary form in intergenerational relations, wherein, for example, adult children take care of ageing parents who took care of them in their childhoods, or young children are dependent on nurturing adults, who, in turn, receive the company of the children and the joys of emotional bonds and affection. This dependence can be seen generally in social life, mutual support, sharing and trust or in negative phenomena, such as alienation, distrust and hate.

Cultural anthropologists have considered reciprocity as an adaptive mechanism that supports survival. According to Matt Ridley (1998, p. 249), reciprocity in society is an inevitable part of our instincts. Humans are predisposed to distinguish the trustworthy from the treacherous, learn how to cooperate, commit to being trustworthy, earn a good reputation and exchange goods and information. The social or symbolic dimensions of the concept of reciprocity can be defined by Maritta Törrönen's (2015) idea of a threefold concept that demands a sense of belonging to a community, legitimisation of one's existence and actions by society, and recognition by other people. Recognition and belonging create positive bonds between people, and legitimisation is a collective bargain to feel justified in existing as a person (Törrönen 2015, p. 82). These elements are highly relevant in social work with children and families. This definition is in harmony with Pierre Bourdieu's (1984) idea of social capital.

Törrönen (2015, pp. 81–82) emphasises the core of reciprocity as the individual's reciprocal social place and as a concept implying empowerment and mutual sharing. However, child welfare clients may have to struggle to find their places and rights in society. In child welfare contexts, this entails focussing on a child in his or her social relationships. Belonging, as experienced by children, is difficult for adults to understand because children are not always able to verbally express their experiences of bonds and dependencies. The development of children's capacity for contingent reciprocity and altruism towards non-relatives is not well known (House *et al.* 2013).

Family bonds are experienced as 'present or given before and beyond any conscious and deliberate individual act'; hence, family ties are not chosen, and personal relations have a 'given nature' (Torche and Valenzuela 2011, p. 189). Family relations are formed from these original bonds. Personal relations in a family can be viewed in terms of co-presence, memory and reciprocity. Child welfare client families may exhibit problems that disturb the experience of reciprocity, such as in cases of neglect, wherein a parent is unable to take care of a child, respond or even be present. The continuity and routines of secure family life may be disrupted or absent.

We would like to introduce two promising examples of reciprocity-enhancing models that could be used in relationship-based child welfare practice. The first involves working in cooperation with families and parents, seeking to build trust and identifying the signs of safety (Turnell and Edwards 1997, 1999), and the second is the secure-base model devised by Gillian Schofield with Mary Beek (Schofield 2002; Schofield and Beek 2005, 2009). In the signs-of-safety model, the basic idea is that every family has strengths, resources and particular ways of solving problems. These can be called 'signs of safety' (Turnell and Edwards 1999, p. 37), wherein safety is composed of the characteristics of the family. The objective is a partnership wherein a family and parents can understand the shared goal: the child's safety (Turnell and Edwards 1997, 1999). This model has been implemented widely in Australia, North America and Europe (Bunn 2013, p. 7), and on the basis of a retrospective study, this model has changed organisational structure and culture, and contributed to internal changes in practitioners' actions and interactions with families (Salveron *et al.* 2015).

Gillian Schofield and colleagues (2005) have developed the secure-base model, which is an integrated psychosocial model for long-term foster care, emphasising the significance of a secure base in the study Growing Up in Foster Care during 1997–2006 (Schofield and Beek 2009). Schofield *et al.* (2005, pp. 7–8) concisely stated five attachment theory-related developmental goals in terms of the dimensions of caregiving that foster children's development, including promotion of trust and caregiver availability, reflective function, self-esteem, autonomy and family membership. The fundamental idea is that interaction with these dimensions reinforces the experience of a secure base in the child's mind. During adolescence, this entails promoting autonomy while simultaneously providing a safe haven and an ongoing sense of relatedness (Schofield and Beek 2005, 2009, p. 260).

In supporting children, multiple care-related needs have to be given focus, and this secure-base model shows the relatedness of care needs and the dynamics of caregiving in responding to them. The secure-base model promotes family membership and responds to the child's need to belong. The meaning of belonging can be seen as multidimensional and, according to a study by Schofield (2002, p. 267), seems related to the family's solidarity, rituals, relationships, identity and culture. The secure-base model is a reciprocal model for promoting security. It focusses on children's needs but also emphasises interaction and the role of caregivers in responding to security needs. The model pays attention to resource-deficient environments and accords value to the practical tasks of social work without separating these from the psychological aspects of social work practice (Ruch 2005, p. 115).

The models mentioned have proven fruitful contributions to work *with* and *in* relationships. However, there are also critical considerations concerning the transportability of interventions into new contexts and cultures (Sundell and Ferrer-Wreder 2014), for example, into Nordic welfare systems. We need careful implementation of different models and evaluation studies of the implementation processes as well as follow-up of outcomes. Reciprocity as a positive concept and goal fits well with the relationship-oriented and relationship-based models of working with children and families. According to Helen Hingley-Jones and Gillian Ruch (2016, p. 236), the term 'relationship-based practice' has been taken into use only relatively recently within the social work education and practice sector, and there is variation in terms of how it is understood theoretically. Their approach to relationship-based practice is rooted in psychodynamic and systemic theories, as detailed in the following. Our thinking is also committed to these traditions within social work, and we suggest a focus on the development of reciprocal relationships in a family.

Developmental origins of reciprocity and its implications for child welfare

Relationship-based child welfare work requires a sound, research grounded understanding of childhood, child development and parenting. Relationship-based work with children and families can have diverse theoretical roots, including those of psychosocial and psychodynamic origins (Trevithick 2003, p. 164). The attachment theory heritage and its applications in social work are valuable and especially useful in child welfare contexts. The starting point for child welfare work is that 'all children need protective, supportive, and emotionally responsive relationships in order to thrive' (Lawler *et al.* 2011, p. 473). These relationships are embedded in multilayered systemic contexts.

Additionally, relationship-based child welfare work with children, young people and adults demands specific theories and research into the development of basic trust and reciprocity, stemming from psychoanalytic and ethological theories and multidisciplinary research. Taking a psychodynamic perspective, Erik H. Erikson (1950, p. 80) viewed trust as a 'basic sense of faith in the self and others'. Later interpretations of early trust have regarded it as developmental, sensory, prelogical, pervasive and dependent upon sensitive parenting. It influences perceptions of social situations involving risk. The fundamental sense of trust may be influenced by traumatic or otherwise significant experiences, such as abuse or serious illness. Among older children and adults, trust is primarily experienced directly on a conscious level at which feelings of trust and decisions are influenced by immediate trustworthiness cues and past interactions with the trustworthiness of others (Bernath and Feshbach 1995).

Research shows that neonates are prepared for social interaction and capable of shaping their experiences actively. They are able to attend to some features, such as the human face, in their environment and block out unwanted stimulation through inattention. Child-caregiver effects are bidirectional, and remarkable reciprocity and mutuality is seen already at 4–6 weeks of age (Schaffer 1977). Colwyn Trevarthen (1993) has presented the notion of intersubjectivity as an innate pattern of human communication because infants show highly discriminating responses to people in contrast to objects. Caregiver-child interactions are also held to be the crucible for concern for others through expansion of the child's sensitivity to others' emotional states and the internalisation of experiences of a loving adult's empathic care (Zahn-Waxler *et al.* 1992).

Research by social workers James Robertson and Joyce Robertson into children's psychological reactions to separation from their attachment figures influenced John Bowlby's theory on attachment (Bowlby 1969, 1973, 1980). His main concern was the nature and vicissitudes of attachment, the enduring and powerful bond that develops in early life between the growing individual and the caregiver. He rooted his theory in psychoanalytic thinking but replaced its traditional metapsychology with a new paradigm based on developmental psychology and ethology. Mary Ainsworth and her associates (Ainsworth *et al.* 1978) observed mothers' styles of responding to the behaviours of their infants. They noticed that responsive mothers gave their children physical care, emotional communication and affection in clear relation to the children's signals of need. The mother's, father's or other primary caregivers' reciprocal responses are contingent on the child's behaviour-reinforced communication attempts, such as babbling and laughing. Secure attachment takes place when children feel able to rely on their caregivers to address their needs for proximity, emotional support and protection. Responsive caregivers also gave their children enough 'space' when they were playing, crawling or exploring their environment independently.

If the attachment between an infant and a caregiver is anxious-ambivalent, the infant feels separation anxiety when separated from the caregiver and does not feel reassured upon the caregiver's return. Anxious-avoidant attachment can be seen when an infant does not show signs of being distressed when the caregiver leaves and does not show positive emotions when she returns. Disorganised attachment involves a lack of attachment behaviour. Mary Main and Erik Hesse (1990) have postulated that the caregiver of a child whose attachment is disorganised is unpredictably frightening to the child, and the disorganisation is a response to this fear and inconsistency.

Nicola Diamond and Mario Marrone (2003, p. 70) argue that attachment security is a broad concept needing clarification. A child may be securely attached to one caregiver and insecurely attached to another or may be securely or insecurely attached to both. This also suggests that security or insecurity of attachment is reflected in styles of relating and psychological functioning, such as sense of self and self-esteem, which can be assessed independently of security of attachment but may be indirect indicators of it. Attachment theory is continuously evolving, generating new specifications and formulations (Crittenden 1995, Marrone 2014). In the 1980s, the theory was extended to attachments in adults and to intergenerational perspectives (Grossman *et al.* 2005). Robert Kahn and Toni Antonucci (1980) suggest that emotional bonding as well as nurturant and supportive aspects of adult relationships exist, although adult life is also dominated by formalised expectations, obligations and roles. In some families, possibly in connection with parental health or substance abuse issues, children may already adopt caring roles in childhood (Dearden and Becker 2004).

The effects of neglect (Smith and Fong 2004) and maltreatment on children and their behaviour in new relationships have also been studied from an attachment theory perspective (e.g. Kaufman and Cicchetti 1989). Children with experiences of maltreatment tend to have a cautious and reserved stance toward others and not be very trusting (Bugental 1993). They may also be traumatised. Insecurely attached children may lack coherent strategies for regulating close relations, which also creates a challenge for professional work. Michael J. Lawler *et al.* (2011) have presented intervention-based models for approaching maltreatment by focussing on dyadic relationships between a child and a parent or surrogate parent. They emphasise the parent's attachment orientation, history and internal working models of self and relationships, and the relationship between the intervener and the dyad is viewed as a key component for the intervention.

David Howe (1997, p. 167) uses the expression 'interpersonal environment of children' to include the qualities of relationships between parents and also children's relationships with carers, siblings, other family members and peers. The individual's psychological coherence and competence is related to the relationship history. Howe does not believe that social work is based only on psychological individualism; it has to also consider the broader social and cultural environment of the child and the family. Relationship-based practice should not marginalise the social dimensions of clients' lives (Ruch 2005, p. 119), and the child's social context is pertinent to child welfare. For example, issues of children's rights and social justice are fundamental in child welfare work. Ruch (2005, p. 114) writes about the need for a holistic approach and integrated understanding of the individual-structural causes of social distress. The focus should be on personal relationships within families but also on the families' socioeconomic statuses and contexts, along with the stressors that may affect how children and parents cope. The power of the theoretical approaches is that they aid in understanding the dynamics of reciprocal relationships in families and also aim to understand the complexity of human beings.

The relationships between parents and child welfare social workers

Reciprocity in child welfare work is a multilayered phenomenon. In contrast with reciprocal relationships in other contexts, it is embedded in complicated relationships between social workers and clients, with foster carers, with other professionals and care organisations, and in relationships within client families and their social networks. Children and families may suffer from problems such as stress, financial problems or neglect and maltreatment, which can endanger reciprocal and positive interaction between family members. Also, the conditions for a child's development of trust and reciprocal relationships may not be optimally met in a family in crisis. Lack of reciprocity may be manifested in multiple relationships, and the challenge of child welfare is how to reflect relationships and support parents in building and sustaining reciprocal relationships with their children.

An important ethical question is raised by the ways in which child welfare or public authorities can expect parents to take good care of their children. From the reciprocity angle, becoming a child welfare client does not entail an equal relationship involving sharing, exchange and giving and receiving something. Those families who have used child welfare services may or may not have a history of seeking and requesting help from relatives and services, which may create obstacles for engaging with service systems. Research identifies several reasons in terms of obstacles to seeking or receiving help. Individual linked factors in withdrawal or resistance may arise from fear, information access problems, attitudes to help-seeking, misconceptions about services, communication difficulties, family members' hostility to interventions and day-to-day stresses and complexities (Cortis *et al.* 2009). Child welfare may detect complex dependencies and hidden elements, such as family secrets. According to Carol Smart (2011, p. 551), all types of family secrets have effects on relationships. In particular, secrets related to reproduction or sexuality have the power to reconfigure family relationships. It is also important to acknowledge that people may not engage with services because the services are inappropriate to their needs.

The term 'hard-to-reach families' has been applied to people who do not readily receive services. Synonyms include 'hidden populations', 'fragile families' and those with 'complex needs'. Among the adjectives used are 'under-served', 'socially excluded', 'vulnerable' and 'high-risk'. Certain ethnic or minority groups/communities may also be less likely to access services (Boag-Munroe and Evangelou 2012, pp. 211–212). Social, economic and cultural structures may cause difficulties in ensuring services and interventions for all families, and service providers may fail to cater to some families' needs. Finally, 'service-resistant' highlights the responsibility of individuals to receive services (Cortis *et al.* 2009, p. 3). Studies of hard-to-reach families have enhanced the awareness of difficulties in understanding families and their ways of living. Engagement issues with all families should be addressed, no matter their backgrounds, to enable discussion or intervention in relationships. The question of whether or not there is a right to resist participation requires discussion and ethical consideration.

Engagement can be defined from involvement, cooperation and participation standpoints. According to James Gladstone *et al.* (2014, p. 56), worker and parent engagement correlate in child welfare casework. It is a reciprocal process between service providers and social workers and the children's families. Engagement equates to processes facilitating involvement in services (Cortis *et al.* 2009, p. 3). Studies of casework skills suggest that relationship-building skills are necessary but not sufficient: Skills that support a collaborative relationship and anti-oppressive approach are also needed. Parents must be included in planning; social workers have to be caring and supportive, and they must appreciate parents' efforts and achievements (Gladstone *et al.* 2014).

When parents struggle with many challenges in private family lives, they do not always readily reveal their life situations to child welfare workers. Parental engagement with child welfare services is a prerequisite to relationship-based work and a predictor of child welfare outcomes. Dendy Platt (2012, p. 142) defines parental engagement in child welfare contexts as the 'mutual, purposeful, behavioural and interactional participation of parent(s) and/or carers in services and interventions provided by social work and other relevant agencies with the aim of achieving positive outcomes'. The relationships between child welfare workers and children and parents are not reciprocal in the sense of equal sharing and mutual exchange nor is this the ultimate goal in child welfare work. The literature and models (e.g. the integrated model of parental engagement; see Platt 2012) help child welfare workers to understand clients' social and psychological backgrounds and how willing and able they are to work with child welfare services. People are not always rational; conscious and unconscious affective dimensions both enrich and complicate human relationships, including professional relationships. Social workers must be able to reflect on their skills and the uses of self and relationships through which interventions are channelled (Ruch 2011).

Relationships with parents who struggle with daily problems do not exist in a vacuum. The family context, the services context and all the child- and case-related issues have an impact in terms of how child welfare workers work with parents in child welfare. Also, parents' previous experiences influence their willingness to work with public authorities as legally mandated decision-makers.

In cases in which the child is placed in out-of-home care, the challenge is to support relationships between child and biological parents, to maintain their relationships and interaction during the placement. A child has a right to safe and continuous reciprocal relationships and environment that supports well-being and healthy development, whether he/she is in the parental home or in out-of-home care.

Building up reciprocal relations between children and child welfare workers

Relationship-based social work and research involving vulnerable children and sensitive concerns poses ethical, practical and emotional challenges for children and professionals. Child welfare social workers meet children and young people in various contexts, for several purposes, to safeguard the children's safety, stability and well-being. Encounters with social workers involve many kinds of experiences and meanings for children and social workers. Also, children may possess knowledge that no one else does, which may lead to hasty information-seeking from children.

Previous qualitative studies based on interviews with children and social workers (e.g. Bell 2002, Pölkki *et al.* 2012, Bijleveld *et al.* 2015) show that children hope that social workers will be genuinely interested in them, listen, convey accurate and vital information, and consider the children's opinions and wishes. In our own study (Pölkki *et al.* 2012), a child said, '*A good social worker, she listens to the young person and understands her feelings and if she has some worries, and she can always be contacted*'. The child was astonished when social workers failed to notice the real situation in the family: '*I found it quite foolish that they never grasped that everything was upset down in that household*'. Children also sought sufficient, accurate information about reasons for their placements and plans for their futures. They felt that they were better heard and more able to influence their own affairs after being placed in a foster home than in community-based services. Social workers identified many obstacles to children's participation, many of these connected with shortages in human and organisational resources or their own skills in working with children. They also mentioned children's loyalty to parents and reflected on the influence of personality and lack of support in emotionally burdensome work. These are key aspects in relationship-based work.

What happens in face-to-face encounters between professionals, children and parents is seldom observed, though it is crucial to understanding the dynamics of practice and advancing theoretical knowledge and skills in effective social work. Karen Broadhurst and Claire Mason (2012) have emphasised the value of face-to-face practice today as the use of mediated communications, such as virtual display units, becomes more widespread. They introduce the concept of corporeal co-presence, arguing that it has much to offer social work practitioners.

Drawing on a participant observation-based study of face-to-face encounters between social workers, children and families, Harry Ferguson (2016a) concluded that most children were seen and engaged with in some manner by social workers who attempted to ascertain their well-being and needs. Only in exceptional situations did social workers' practices not meaningfully focus on the children, with the children rendered partially or even totally invisible. Later, Ferguson (2016b) deepened understanding of how and why children become invisible in everyday child protection practice, showing that the practice achieves different degrees of closeness to children and families. In some short- and long-term work, relationships with children were very close and intimate: The children were not only talked to but also hugged, caressed to provide comfort, examined and played with. Children aged four and above were spoken to on their own. Ferguson's work shows that when children are not meaningfully engaged with, the absence of an intimate approach that involves eye-to-eye contact, talk, active listening, play, touch and close observation is most relevant. Hence, he suggests the term 'unheld child' instead of 'invisible child'. Karen Winter and her colleagues (2017) have also demonstrated interesting and helpful strategies, e.g. play, that social workers use in child welfare work with children.

In addition, Ferguson (2016b) has described how social workers have been overcome by the work's emotional intensity and complex interactions with angry, resistant parents and family friends. Workers were additionally affected by organisational culture, time constraints and insufficient support in containing their feelings and thinking clearly. It was difficult to 'keep clients in mind'. Hence, invisible children are those who become 'unthought about' by workers and systems. Child protection professionals experience intense emotions (anxiety, fear, hope, despair and hate), which are projected onto them by clients. Crucial here is whether and how these unavoidable feelings are managed and contained in ways that promote clear thinking. If workers lack containment opportunities (e.g. supervision, discussion with colleagues), links between thoughts and feelings may be broken and professionals may defend themselves against unbearable feelings by detaching physically and emotionally, sometimes even dissociating from those seeking help.

Ganna Van Bijleveld and colleagues (2015) have suggested that the personal relationship between a child and a social worker is among the most important facilitators to participation. Barriers to creating this relationship have been demonstrated by children, case managers and social workers. Professionals have also identified situations wherein children's participation is inappropriate. This objection may stem from the sociocultural image of children as vulnerable and in need of adult protection. Tensions exist between a child's right to participate and be protected. Johanna Hurtig (2006) has analysed professional interpretation frameworks that prevent social workers from asking a child important questions: A child is too vulnerable or even fragile, a child is an inseparable part of the family, a child's loyalty prevents him/her from revealing family issues, and talking about family matters to social workers causes problems for children. These frameworks reveal the complicated dynamics of encounters with children. Child welfare social workers have the interrelated and even conflicting roles and tasks of case workers or counsellors, advocates, partners, assessors of risk or need, care managers and agents of social control (Asquith *et al.* 2005, pp. 2–3, Winter 2009).

Children's rights have been promoted in many ways over recent decades; however, a child may be dependent and powerless in his/her relationship to the social worker. The more a child is at risk, the more power the social worker may use in decisions that influence the life and future of the child. The social worker has the responsibility to promote the participation of the child in child welfare processes and, in its deepest sense, in his/her own life.

Discussion

The discussion surrounding relationship-based child welfare work is extensive and impossible to review exhaustively. A lot of sound theorising on the relationship-based approach already exists. The attachment framework and a psychosocial orientation have been strongly present in the field of child welfare (Howe 1997, Lawler *et al.* 2011), and good models for working with children and parents exist. Research demonstrates a need to reflect on the dynamics and complexities of clients and relationships, which necessitates a holistic and systemic (Ruch 2005; see also Trevithick 2003) or integrated model for helping families with problems (e.g. Platt 2012) and recognition-oriented approaches (Turney 2012). When assessing the child's best interest, reciprocity is not yet widely theorised upon. We argue that reciprocity may offer a theoretical basis for relationship-based child welfare.

Since the Convention on the Rights of the Child (1989) introduced the three hard P's – protection, participation and provision – into international discussions, much effort has been made in child and family policies in many countries, including Finland. Reciprocity is in some way crystallised in principles of safety, permanence and well-being in international conventions and child welfare literature. Professional and public awareness of vulnerable children has increased in recent years, and preventative measures have been developed. In the Nordic welfare system, collaboration between early educators and personnel at maternity and child health clinics is a resource in meeting the needs of almost all children under school age (Pölkki and Vornanen 2015). It is still worth asking whether child welfare professionals really understand the child or young person in her/his context, understand the dynamics of reciprocal relationships and are able to work intensively in and with the relationships around the developing person.

The problems in a family are not always temporary crises; rather, they may be rooted in family history, poverty or poor neighbourhoods, and they may develop and escalate over a long period of time. Thus, there is reason to reflect on whether the reciprocal and safe relationships in a family have been endangered. From the perspective of reciprocity, the assessment in child welfare should focus on the relationship history, the intensity and quality of the emotional relationships, and whether good care is provided. Reciprocal relationships are crucial to a child's feeling of being recognised and to his/ her development of subjectivity and self-esteem. During the primary social-isation process and in encounters with professionals, issues concerning so-ciety's legitimation of one's existence and actions are relevant. The concept of reciprocity strengthens the understanding of belonging, recognition and legitimation in child welfare.

As presented in the preceding chapters, there are several prerequisites and obstacles in reciprocal and relationship-based child welfare work with chil-dren, young people and adults. There is also increasing information on the essential elements of working models, which are helpful – at least in some contexts. For example, the two models presented, the signs-of-safety model and the secure-base model, emphasise working in and with relationships for the security of the child. The quality of relationships and contact with child welfare services is crucial: It either promotes or inhibits the possibility of working in a relationship. The initial engagement is tested during work with a family. Child welfare literature presents several types of approaches to relationship-based child welfare work. These models, we argue, are relevant for focussing on the dynamics of reciprocal relationships in child welfare client families and can offer practical input for getting various kinds of fam-ilies with children engaged in working on relationships.

A child and his/her parents meet child welfare social workers who they do not know, and they are expected to trust them with their personal and pri-vate issues. This challenges the development and use of relationship-based working models in child welfare. First encounters are significant: They cre-ate the basis for further work and additional assistance processes. The en-gagement of parents may either contribute to or prevent the child welfare social worker's ability to effectively help children. The sides of the triangle between child, parents and social worker can have different demands, de-pending on what kinds of support or intervention the child and family need. When the reciprocal relationship is weak between a child and a parent, stronger support may be needed from the social network and from the child welfare social worker who is coordinating support for the child. Situations involving impending danger may be difficult to detect in the absence of a trusting relationship with the child.

The relationship-based approach to child welfare requires a sound knowl-edge basis that consists of knowledge about theories on childhood, child development and social work as well as practical knowledge. We emphasise the knowledge production of children and parents as well as the engagement of parents in supporting reciprocal and emotionally responsive relationships. Child welfare social work always entails working with and in relationships, even though social workers' orientations and approaches may vary. We suggest reflecting on current practices by focussing on the working relationship between professionals, parents and children, and special theoretical models for working more intensively. Psychosocial and therapeutic elements are involved in work with vulnerable clients in vulnerable contexts. Child welfare social workers need good practical and counselling skills, but psychotherapeutic services should also be available to support clients.

Our conclusion is that a focus on reciprocity in child welfare is important, not only in tackling the risks associated with child neglect and maltreatment but also in obtaining social capital during childhood. The question of reciprocity is crucial for the development of social capital, particularly where problems are severe and long-term. This has implications for both child welfare research and for the development of relationship-based practices.

References

Ainsworth, M. D. S., Blehar, M. C., Waters, E. and Wall, S., 1978. *Patterns of attachment: A psychological study of the strange situation.* Hillsdale, NJ: Erlbaum.

Asquith, S., Clark, C. and Waterhouse, I., 2005. *The role of the social worker in the 21st century: A literature Review.* Edinburgh: Scottish Executive.

Bell, M., 2002. Promoting children's rights through the use of relationship. *Child & Family Social Work*, 7, 1–11.

Bernath, S. and Feshbach, N. D., 1995. Children's trust: Theory, assessment, development, and research directions. *Applied and Preventive Psychology*, 4, 1–19.

Boag-Munroe, G. and Evangelou, M., 2012. From hard to reach to how to reach: A systematic review of the literature on hard-to-reach families. *Research Papers in Education*, 27 (2), 209–239.

Bourdieu, P., 1984/1979. *Distinction: A social critique of the judgment of taste.* Cambridge, MA: Harvard University Press.

Bowlby, J., 1969. *Attachment and loss, vol. 1: Attachment*, 2nd ed. London: Penguin Books.

Bowlby, J., 1973. *Attachment and loss, vol. 2: Separation.* London: Hogarth Press.

Bowlby, J., 1980. *Attachment and loss, vol. 3: Loss, sadness and depression.* London: Hogarth Press.

Broadhurst, K. and Mason, C., 2012. Social work beyond the VDU: Foregrounding co-presence in situated practice – why face-to-face practice matters. *British Journal of Social Work Advance Access*, published 5 September 2012.

Bugental, D. B., 1993. Perceived control and child abuse. *Scientist*, 45, 294–304.

Bunn, A. 2013. Signs of safety in England. An NSPCC commissioned report of the signs of safety model in child protection. NSPCC. https://www.nspcc.org.uk/globalassets/documents/research-reports/signs-safety-england.pdf [Accessed 13 October 2016].

Child Welfare Act. 2007. Unofficial translation. Ministry of social affairs and health, Finland. http://www.finlex.fi/en/laki/kaannokset/2007/en20070417.pdf [Accessed 15 May 2016].

Cortis, N., Katz, I. and Patulny, R., 2009. Engaging hard-to-reach families and children. Canberra: Australian Government Department of Families, Housing, Community Services and Indigenous Affairs. https://www.dss.gov.au/sites/default/files/documents/op26.pdf [Accessed 13 October 2016].

Crittenden, P. M., 1995. Attachment and psychopathology. In: S. Goldberg, R. Muir and J. Kerr (eds.) *John Bowlby's attachment theory: Historical, clinical and social significance,* (pp. 367–406), NY: Analytical Press.

Dearden, C. and Becker, S., 2004. Young carers in the UK: The 2004 Report. London: Carers UK.

Diamond, N. and Marrone, M., 2003. *Attachment and intersubjectivity.* London: Whurr.

Diekmann, A., 2004. The power of reciprocity: Fairness, reciprocity, and stakes in variants of the dictator game. *Journal of Conflict Resolution,* 48 (4), 487–505.

Erikson, E. H., 1950. Childhood and society. New York: W.W. Norton & Company, Inc.

European Convention on Human Rights. European Court of Human Rights. Council of Europe. http://www.echr.coe.int/Documents/Convention ENG.pdf [Accessed 15 May 2016].

Ferguson, H., 2016a. What social workers do in performing child protection work: Evidence from research into face-to-face practice. *Child & Family Social Work,* 21, 283–294.

Ferguson, H., 2016b. How children become invisible in child protection work: Findings from research into day-to-day social work practice. *British Journal of Social Work Advance Access,* published 30 June 2016.

Gilbert, N., ed., 1997. *Combatting child abuse: International perspectives and trends.* New York: Oxford University Press.

Gilbert, N., Parton, N. and Skiveness, M., 2011. *Child protection systems: International trends and orientations.* New York: Oxford University Press.

Gladstone, J., *et al.,* 2014. Understanding worker–parent engagement in child protection casework. *Children and Youth Services Review,* 44, 56–64.

Grossman, K. E., Grossmann, K. and Waters, E., 2005. *Attachment from infancy to adulthood.* New York: Guilford Press.

Hearn, J., *et al.,* 2004. What is child protection? Historical and methodological issues in comparative research on lastensuojelu/child protection. *International Journal of Social Welfare,* 13 (1), 28–41.

Hingley-Jones, H. and Ruch, G., 2016. 'Stumbling though'? Relationship-based social work practice in austere times, *Journal of Social Work Practice,* 30 (3), 235–248.

House, B., Henrich, J., Sarecka, B. and Silk, J. B. 2013. *Evolution and human behaviour,* 24 (1), 86–93.

Howe, D. 1997. Psychosocial and relationship-based theories for child and family social work: Political philosophy, psychology and welfare practice. *Child and Family Social Work,* 2, 161–169.

Hurtig, J., 2006. Lasten tieto sosiaalityön haasteena (Children's knowledge as a challenge for social work). In: J. H. Forsberg, A. Ritala-Koskinen and M. Törrönen (eds.) *Lapset ja sosiaalityö. (Children and social work).* pp. 167–193. Jyväskylä: PS-kustannus.

Kahn, R. L. and Antonucci, T. C., 1980. Convoys over the life course: Attachment, roles, and social support. In: P. B. Baltes and O. Brim (eds.) *Life-span development and behavior*, 3, 253–268. New York: Academic Press.

Kaufman, J. and Cicchetti, D., 1989. Effects of maltreatment in school-age children's socio-emotional development: Assessments in a day-camp setting. *Developmental Psychology*, 25, 516–524.

Lawler, M. J., Shaver, P. R. and Goodman, G. S., 2011. Toward relationship-based child welfare services. *Children and Youth Services Review*, 33, 473–480.

Main, M. and Hesse, E., 1990. Parents' unresolved traumatic experiences are related to infant disorganized attachment status: Is frightened and/or frightening parental behavior the linking mechanism? In: M. Greenberg, D. Cicchetti, and M. Cummings (eds.) *Attachment in the Preschool Years*. Chicago: Chicago University Press.

Marrone, M. 2014/1998. *Attachment and interaction*. 2nd ed. London: Jessica Kingsley Publishers.

Molm, L. D., 2010. The structure of reciprocity. *Social Psychological Quarterly*, 73 (2), 119–131.

O'Leary, P., Tsui, M. S. and Ruch, G., 2013. The boundaries of the social work relationship revisited: Towards a connected, inclusive and dynamic conceptualisation. *British Journal of Social Work*, 43, 135–153.

Platt, D., 2012. Understanding parental engagement with child welfare services: An integrated model. *Child and Family Social Work*, 17, 138–148.

Pölkki, P., 1992. Is the voice of children at risk heard in the Finnish child welfare system. In: P.-L. Heiliö, E. Lauronen and M. Bardy (eds.) *Politics of childhood and children at risk: provision—protection—participation*. Helsinki: Stakes, 91–93.

Pölkki, P., Vornanen, R., Pursiainen, M. and Riikonen, M., 2012. Children's participation in child protection processes as experienced by foster children and social workers. *Child Care in Practice*, 18 (2), 107–125.

Pölkki, P. L. and Vornanen, R., 2015. Role and success of Finnish early childhood education and care in supporting child welfare clients: perspectives from parents and professionals. *Early Childhood Education Journal*, 44, 581–594.

Pölkki, P. L., Vornanen, R. and Colliander, R., 2016. Critical factors of intensive family work connected with positive outcomes for child welfare clients. *The European Journal of Social Work*. doi: 10.1080/13691457.2015.1137868 (published online first), http://dx.doi.org/10.1080/13691457.2015.1137868.

Pösö, T., 2011. Combatting child abuse in Finland. In: N. Gilbert, N. Parton and M. Skivenes (eds.) *Child protection systems: international trends and orientations*. New York: Oxford University Press, 112–130.

Ridley, M., 1998. *The origins of virtue*. UK: Penguin UK.

Ruch, G., 2005. Relationship based practice and reflective practice: Holistic approaches to contemporary child care social work. *Child and Family Social Work*, 10, 111–123.

Ruch, G., 2011. Where have all the feelings gone? Developing reflective and relationship-based management in child-care social work. *British Journal of Social Work*, 42 (7), 1315–1332.

Ruch, G. and Julkunen, I., (eds.) 2016. *Relationship-based research in social work. Understanding practice research*. London: Jessica Kingsley Publishers.

Salveron, M., Bromfield, L., Kirika, C., Simmons, J., Murphy, T. and Turnell, A., 2015. 'Changing the way to do child protection': The implementation of signs of safety within the Western Australia department for child protection and family support. *Children and Youth Services Review*, 48, 126–139.

Schaffer, R., 1977. *Mothering*. Cambridge, MA: Harvard University Press.

Schofield, G., 2002. The significance of a secure base: A psychosocial model of long-term foster care. *Child and Family Social Work*, 7, 259–272.

Schofield, G. and Beek, M., 2005. Providing a secure base: Parenting children in long-term foster family care. *Attachment & Human Development*, 7 (19), 3–25.

Schofield, G. and Beek, M., 2009. Growing up in foster care: Providing a secure base through adolescence. *Child and Family Social Work*, 14, 255–266.

Smart, C. 2011. Families, secrets and memories. *Sociology*, 45, 539–553.

Smith, M. and Fong, R., 2004. *The children of neglect: When no one cares*. New York: Brunner-Routledge.

Social Welfare Act 2014/1301. Ministry of Social Affairs and Health, Finland. http://stm.fi/en/social-and-health-services/legislation [Accessed 15 May 2016].

STM 2013. Toimiva lastensuojelu. Selvitysryhmän loppuraportti. (A national committee report on child welfare in Finland by the Ministry of Social Affairs and Health) Sosiaali- ja terveysministeriön raportteja ja muistioita 19/2013.

Sundell, K. and Ferrer-Wreder, L., 2014. The transportability of empirically supported interventions. In: A. Shlonsky and R. Benbenishty (eds.) *From evidence to outcomes in child welfare. An international reader*. Oxford: Oxford University Press, 41–58.

Torche, F. and Valenzuela, E., 2011. Trust and reciprocity: A theoretical distinction of the sources of social capital. *European Journal of Social Theory*, 14 (2), 181–198.

Törrönen, M., 2015. Toward a theoretical framework for social work—reciprocity: The symbolic justification of existence. *Journal of Social Work Values and Ethics*, 12 (2), 77–87.

Trevarthen, C., 1993. The self born in intersubjectivity. The psychology of an infant communicating. In: U. Neisser (ed.) *The perceived self: Ecological and interpersonal sources of self-knowledge*. New York: Cambridge University Press, 121–173.

Trevithick, P., 2003. Effective relationship-based practice: A theoretical exploration. *Journal of Social Work Practice*, 17 (2), 163–176.

Turnell, A. and Edwards, S., 1997. Aspiring to partnership: The signs of safety approach to child protection. *Child Abuse Review*, 6, 176–190.

Turnell, A. and Edwards, S., 1999. *Signs of safety: A solution and safety oriented approach to child protection casework*. New York: W. W. Norton & Company.

Turney, D., 2012. A relationship-based approach to engaging involuntary clients: The contribution of recognition theory. *Child and Family Social Work*, 17, 149–159.

van Bijleveld, G. G., Dedding, C. W. W. and Bunders-Aelen, J. E. G., 2015. Children's and young people's participation within child welfare and child protection services. A state-of-the-art review. *Child and Family Social Work*, 20, 129–138.

Winter, K., 2009. Relationships matter: The problem and prospects for social workers' relationships with young children in care. *Child and Family Social Work*, 14, 450–460.

Winter, K., Cree, V., Hallett, S., Hadfield, M., Ruch, G., Morrison, F. and Holland, S., 2017. Exploring communication between social workers, children and young people. *British Journal of Social Work*, 47 (5), 1–18.

Wood, A., 2001. The origins of family systems work: Social workers' contributions to the development of family theory and practice. *Australian Social Work*, 54 (3), 15–29.

Zahn-Waxler, C, Radke-Yarrow, M., Wagner, E. and Chapman, M., 1992. Development of concern for others. *Developmental Psychology*, 28, 126–136.

Part III

Reciprocity

Methodological and
educational issues

8 Reciprocity with graduate students fostered through creativity

Tuula Heinonen

Introduction

In many universities around the world, the work of academic advisors with their social work students is often constructed as a one-to-one relationship in which an expert guides the novice and helps her or him to become socialised to the academic environment of learning and achievement. Geoff Gurr (2001) maintains that this time-honoured method in graduate education is seen as a key to success for students. It is generally a feature in higher-level education, for example, in academic advising and supervision in Canadian universities, including the University of Manitoba, where the author is located. In Canada, graduate social work education is generally offered in universities that have long histories and conventions in academic advising. In such situations, reciprocity may be less a priority in academic guidance and supervision than motivating and guiding the student to succeed in their studies and complete their programs. Thus, the roles of advisor and student could be compared to those of expert and novice. However, when reciprocity is introduced as a component part of academic advising and supervision, and graduate students are encouraged to actively engage in reflexive shared processes with their advisors, a different relationship can result. Outcomes of such relationships can include collaborative activities, such as discussion about conceptual topics, joint research and co-authorship of publications (see Halse and Bansel 2012). Complementary methods that are suited for use in social work-advisor relationships across educational settings internationally may also be introduced. This example is an alternative method for the purpose of enhancing reflection and fostering a climate of reciprocity for learning between student and advisor.

This chapter looks at the role that creative methods can play in enhancing the quality of learning and the process of engagement in graduate studies in which both advisor and student participate. The author introduced a mixed media art exercise that engaged graduate students in reflecting on the past year of studies and creating a visual depiction of their experiences and impressions into their annual reviews of their academic progress over the year (Heinonen 2015). With their artwork, students included short descriptions and comments about the art and its meaning to them. After receiving the students' artwork and narratives, the author, as advisor, produced for each of them a reply using visual depiction and text. This method is referred to as 'response art' (Fish 2008) and is drawn from expressive arts supervision to encourage practitioner expression and reflection and dialogue with supervisees. In this exercise, reciprocity was fostered, resulting in new insights for both and a more effective and enhanced advisor-graduate student relationship.

Background and context

I have found graduate supervision to be an art that is shaped over time and draws from one's professional and personal values and beliefs, educational vision and practice principles and orientation. For many educators, it is a stimulating, challenging and rewarding experience to work with graduate students and see them develop academically and professionally. Students have also been my teachers, helping me to reflect on my supervision practice and to hone my skills as a mentor, guide, collaborator and advocate for their graduate success.

Having completed several years of study in art therapy and applied my learning in various group work settings and activities, I wanted to introduce it into the supervision of graduate students in social work. I had experienced the arts as a vehicle for reflection, expression and change, and I benefited from learning about uses of visual art as a vehicle for my own professional development. Further, I had enjoyed a reciprocal relationship with my art therapy practice supervisor. These experiences contributed to my ideas on integrating arts-based methods into student supervision. I saw enormous potential in arts-based approaches and reciprocal learning in supervision and decided to make use of visual art methods in my supervision work with graduate students. I observed during this process how reciprocity was fostered through reflection and discussion in a co-creative process between the graduate students and me. Of course, reciprocity in relationships between students and advisors can occur in other ways, such as through collaborating on projects, co-teaching, and more. Here, I am focussing only on reciprocity that results from the practice of art-making in the context of a supervisory relationship. Although there has been a resurgence of arts-based methods in social work practice and research, writing on the use of such methods in graduate supervisory experience is rare (Barrett and Hussey 2015). There is a need for further exploration of the potential contributions (and limitations) of arts-based methods with graduate students and the evaluation of such methods. Research on both processes and outcomes' making use of qualitative (narratives from both students and supervisors) and quantitative (timely graduation and successful grades) methods could be helpful.

In an effort to add a participative and more reciprocal process in the annual progress review of graduate students, I initiated a parallel exercise that made use of collage and mixed media art exercises. I use some excerpts and examples from my own response art (Fish 2008) for the students to illustrate my responses to their art and narratives during annual progress reviews that were to be completed by supervisors with their students. Finally, I summarise the experience of reciprocity in these experiences and the potential for expressive arts integration to foster reciprocal relationships in social work supervision.

Graduate student supervision

Educators in professional programs, such as social work, conduct graduate student supervision as part of their university teaching work. They regularly meet with their graduate students to discuss topics such as student progress, programme timelines, feedback on written work, suggestions for additional inquiry and reading as well as concepts and theories relevant to students' research topics. These meetings (held annually or more often) usually occur in the supervisor's office, last about an hour and generally consist of a review of checklists related to courses completed, objectives met and timelines followed. The completion of the form is important as it enables the student to progress to the next year of academic study. When the student's progress requires it, such as due to a failed course, need for a leave from studies or an extension of time to complete the program, another meeting is called to discuss the situation, and forms are filled out, prepared and processed for the University. Students tend to see these meetings as hoops they are required to jump through for the University so that they can continue their studies. For the University, the completed forms help in assessing progress and decisions to be taken regarding the student's situation and needs.

Administrative policies and procedures in universities tend to be focussed on accountability in supervising graduate students, and these are expected to be followed by academic supervisors 'through formal, structured, cognitive transmission of knowledge from instructor to learner' (Halse 2011, p. 58). Meetings with graduate students are predicated on a model of good supervision involving transmission of information from supervisor to student.

With mature (adult) students, many of whom have significant professional experience, the supervisory relationship tends to be more collegial; The supervisor and student learn from one another, and a reciprocal style is suited. The supervisor, as an adult educator, makes use of adult education principles and methods to help students draw from their own experiences and construct their own knowledge (Knowles *et al.* 2015). However, the shared interaction and collaboration process in supervision, which significantly contributes to student progress, cannot easily be measured. What is missed, according to Christine Halse (2011, p. 558), is 'the interdependent relationship between the learner, learning and learning context.' As in the classroom, mature social work students learn best through methods that are centred on student interests and relevance to their work and experiences.

Thus, it is important to acknowledge and draw upon their accomplishments and the significant years of work, education and life experience brought into their university studies. Facilitation of learning that is outside conventional frames of knowledge acquisition can be useful. To this end, experiential methods that draw on creative and intuitive knowledge can add to and enrich graduate students' supervision experiences by including the whole person (Coulshed 1993, McArdle *et al.* 2013, Mulder and Dull 2014, Barrett and Hussey 2015).

Reciprocity in supervision

A feature of satisfactory human relationships is positive reciprocity, which takes the form of giving and receiving, sharing and mutual respect. One person's positive deed for another usually encourages the receiver of the good deed to reciprocate in some way to acknowledge or return the favour. In relation to workplace interaction, Bram Buunk *et al.* (1993) refer to social exchange as a feature in reciprocal relationships. In academic supervision, reciprocity is a professional component of the supervisory relationship (Halse 2011); however, it does not mean equality in the relationship. Supervisors do have a position of power over their graduate students, which can be difficult for the student whose work is subjected to critical scrutiny, for example, in marked-up drafts indicating further revision.

Reciprocity is important in social work relationships in which clients and social workers agree that both will expend time and energy working on activities to reach a desired goal. The social worker's genuineness, respect, care, commitment and regard for the client usually result in a positive response from the client. As with client-social work relationships, social work supervisor-supervisee relationships often involve some degree of reciprocity as students and academic advisors develop the terms and expectations of their relationships. For masters and doctoral students, teaching and supervision offer the possibility of interactive discussion and a greater reciprocity between students and educators to enhance learning for both. Veronica Coulshed (1993) states that 'capacity for higher reasoning and critical reflectivity will develop' (p. 6) at the graduate studies level.

Reflection, an important skill in social work student-advisor engagement, is essential in learning from the work done with people and the range of issues they bring. Employing a questioning and open attitude about one's application of theories in practice is important to learning in social work. Supervision, therefore, needs to foster graduate students' capacities and knowledge of self for effective application of theory to the practice of professional social work (Bernard and Goodyear 2004). Academic supervisors would do well to give their students sufficient to explore and present ideas about what they think they did well and what they have concerns about regarding their work. However, for this to occur and for any reciprocity to develop, trust in the relationship is prerequisite.

Christine Halse and Peter Bansel (2012, p. 384) claim that the learning alliance of a student and supervisor relationship is characterised by 'a cooperative endeavour of reciprocal responsibilities and obligations.' In a humanist approach, a reciprocal relationship also includes a facilitative process of student mentorship by supervisors (Cassidy 2009). Consistent with this approach is the facilitation of reflection methods that generate insights and new perspectives for graduate students' studies.

Supervisory relationships with graduate students tend to be more collegial and facilitative due to their different needs and interests as compared to those with undergraduate students. Reciprocity can be more easily developed in graduate student supervision due to the sustained process, which often involves flexible structures, divergent understandings and redundancy in interactions with students (Kalin *et al.* 2009).

In Canadian society, characterised by great ethnocultural diversity and cross-cultural interaction, supervisory relationships often need to be developed across cultures. In such a context, respect, openness and curiosity about fostering effective communication and meaningful guidance are required of academic advisors (Acker 2011). Different expectations of what graduate supervision comprises may exist and need to be discussed and negotiated. Procedures and expectations for supervision of graduate students provide a structure in the university setting for such relationships; however, given each student's unique experience, academic interests and learning needs, space is required to accommodate differences.

There is no doubt that graduate student-advisor relationships are not always successful. Mismatched interpersonal styles and differing needs and expectations can create difficulties. Power differences may be at the root of some of the problems, particularly when students perceive little opportunity to negotiate the content and format of supervisory sessions. In such cases, students may take longer than normal to complete their studies (Murphy 2009). When promoting and practising reciprocity in supervisory relationships, it is important for supervisors to be aware of boundary issues that can lead to expectations that are inappropriate or to relationships similar to those between a therapist and client (Harrison and Grant 2015).

The arts in graduate supervision

Supervision is important for graduate students to progress in their work. Creative methods in supervision can add further depth and meaning that is less often achieved in the supervisory process. Educators have observed benefits from integrating creative methods into teaching and/or supervision as these can enable students to express their ideas and experiences in a visual and/or expressive way (e.g. Walton 2012, Mulder and Dull 2014). Creative methods can also provide new perspectives for academic supervisors, who use arts-based expression as a means of reflection on what they learn from their students and about themselves in the supervisory process (Wehbi 2009). Halse and Bansel (2012) note that using the brain's intuitive and creative parts can offer students a deep and satisfying means of understanding and discussing their work in a student-advisor relationship in which reciprocity is featured. Further, creating artwork as part of the supervision process can be seen 'as a constructivist endeavour, one that requires active participation, invites reflection, and has the capacity to promote deep insights and self-awareness' (Deaver and Shiflett 2011, p. 268). Creative processes represent the highest level of thinking and can advance theoretical analysis and innovation (Simmons and Daley 2013). Expressive arts methods in student supervision can offer a means for students to reflect on their growth and learning over a period of time. Supervisors can make use of such opportunities to address what they have observed and understood in relation to the students' comments (Newsome, Henderson and Veach 2005). Reciprocal reflection may lead to innovative ideas and insights for research or writing when fostered through arts-based exercises that involve both student and advisor. This takes place when the artwork created by the students becomes the focus of discussion, and students are valued as 'the makers of their own knowledge' (McAuliffe 2000).

Creative arts can offer the supervisor and student methods such as storytelling, collage-making, drawing, poetry and photography as complementary methods in the supervisory process. Educators in social work and other professions have seen the benefits for students who draw from their own creative skills (e.g. Walton 2012, McArdle *et al.* 2013, Mulder and Dull 2014). Creative methods can offer rich resources that generate useful insights for students. Arts-informed supervision activities enable the sharing of metaphors, impressions and symbolic images, which illustrate and illuminate beliefs, traditions, values and practices. Art-making in graduate supervision allows for expression and meaning-making in which students can feel heard, validated and appreciated. These practices can be powerful and can imbue the supervisory experience with great depth. Faculty members may thus find it beneficial to apply arts-informed methods as they work with graduate students (Keddell 2011, Hughes 2012, Huss 2012, Konopik and Cheung 2012, Moxley *et al.* 2012, Walton 2012, Desyallas and Sinclair 2014, Mulder and Dull 2014).

Adult students bring their life experiences, infused with their own unique meanings, to the supervision relationship (Shor 1992, Coulshed 1993). Their knowledge and experiences are important resources that add to the synthesis of concepts and theories learned in graduate studies. They can also offer a wealth of material for discussion during supervision. Sharing and discussing material that includes the adult student's knowledge and experiences with the academic supervisor can generate a climate of reciprocity in the relationship, with the supervisor participating as well.

The arts convey powerful and evocative messages to both the creator and audience. Further, restorative, healing and empowering effects can result from the use of music, art and other creative methods. Currently, the resurgence of the arts in social work practice, inquiry and education is apparent, and many authors have published works that reflect a focus on the use of arts-based methods as a complement or sole approach (e.g. Coholic *et al.* 2009, Mulder and Dull 2014, Bonnycastle and Bonnycastle 2015, Conrad and Sinner 2015, Sinding and Barnes 2015).

Use of collage in graduate student supervision

Developing a collage is an open-ended project because it 'represents the practice at a particular moment: Its form and content reflect the juxtaposition of individual ideas, realms of thought, texts, images, and other creative works, and the conversation that develops between them' (Vaughan 2003, p. 41). Collage is a useful creative method for many people because it does not require artistic skill at manipulation of paint, ink, pencils, crayons or other common art supplies. It is accessible and less intimidating for many who do not see themselves as artists.

The potential of one visual arts media – collage – as a creative method can 'communicate thoughts, concepts and allows the learner to further explore connection between concepts and ideas' (Simmons and Daley 2013, p. 4). A collage exercise invites the person creating it to find, select and arrange images, words and ephemera to represent experiences, processes and meanings in concrete or abstract ways. Images placed on a collage can represent something else, such as a bird that is used as a metaphor for freedom. Only the person who has created the collage will be able to describe the meanings in the different elements, the connections between them and the collage as a whole (Butler-Kisber 2010).

A method referred to as response art (Fish 2008) enabled me to respond to the artwork and accounts that the graduate students provided. It was a way for me to provide feedback and affirm what they expressed to me. The response art was used as a way of reciprocating for the art and accounts that the students had given to me. It was part of the process of supervision that occurred between the students and me in 2014–2015, when an art exercise was integrated into graduate student supervision. This art exercise was conducted in conjunction with the annual progress reviews that I held with each graduate student.

In this process, the social work students I supervised were invited to participate in a creative art exercise in which collage and/or mixed art media were used alongside written or verbal accounts that explained what their artwork signified in relation to the question, 'How would you describe both visually and in words your graduate studies experience this year?' The students were told that they were not required to participate and that it was their choice if they wished to do so. Seven graduate students out of twelve participated in 2014, and four out of ten participated in 2015. Some of the same graduate students took part in both 2014 and 2015. Each student produced a piece of art and a short narrative account in which they described the images in their artwork and their significance in relation to the question I had posed. Most students brought or emailed their artwork to me, and we communicated in person, by phone or by email so that they could tell me about their artwork and how it represented what they thought about the past year of their graduate work.

For the collage exercise, I drew from a collection of images compiled from magazines and newspapers over the last five years. The collected images containing interesting colours and textures or different themes, such as machine parts, architecture, people in various activities, roads and pathways and interior and exterior landscapes. I selected from these in my collages for the students.

Within a week, I reviewed what the students had produced and written (or stated) and prepared and sent my own artwork to each of them, along with a written response. I used collage and some mixed media and emailed comments to them to respond to what I had understood from their descriptions of their artwork. Affirmations also comprised a part of my responses to the students as I felt that their significant efforts and commitment to their study goals were important to acknowledge and for the students to hear. I knew that graduate work often occurs in a context of self-discipline and solitude, even when students share what they are working on with others.

Once the students received my comments and artwork, many acknowledged, sometimes in lengthy emails, what the art exercise experience was like for them, what had struck them about the process and what they had learned about themselves. Others wrote shorter emails to thank me for what I sent to them. Some graduate students who did not take part said they did not have time to complete the exercise; a few simply stated that they preferred to discuss their progress in person without any art activity. I considered it important to respect students' wishes about how they wanted to participate in the supervisory review and complied with their preferences.

Selected examples of my response art

For ethical reasons, I do not discuss the students' narrative accounts of their artwork but provide some composite examples of the topics generated. In addition, I focus on my own experience and learning from this creative graduate student supervision exercise. When I first considered the arts-based supervision of graduate students, I knew that it would increase the supervision time needed for me and for each student who took part. This was due to the need to reflect on the art produced by each student and to listen carefully to their words regarding its meaning and significance. It took some time for the students to produce their collages, consider what they wanted to say about them and write these ideas for me. The students described not only the content of their completed pieces but also the process related to thinking and making decisions about what they would include in their artwork. They were required to reflect on and interpret their past year's graduate work and how the art they created reflected their experiences. The graduate students met with me in face-to-face meetings, spoke to me on the telephone or wrote their reflections in email messages. Most enjoyed the art-making and the opportunity to express their ideas in relation to what they had created. Several students wanted to repeat the exercise in the future and told me that they had learned much about achievements they had made in their studies over the course of the year that they would not have realised otherwise. One student said she knew that she was able to focus better on a research idea as a result of the exercise and was eager to start work on a proposal. Five of the graduate students took several hours and considerable care in producing their artwork and were pleased that I responded to it. Two others approached the exercise in a more practical way, seeing it as a different way to describe the work they had done in the last year. For them, the art-making was not particularly stimulating and took only a short time for them to complete.

My responses to the students were as unique as their art pieces, and my interpretations of these pieces had to be tailored uniquely to each individual. I felt honoured to learn what their experiences over the year had meant to them, how they had been challenged by the many demands on their time and energy, and how they had been inspired and motivated by what they had learned and what we shared. I learned from them that it is essential for supervisors to discuss new creative supervision methods with graduate students to help them understand that the rationale for the methods' use is in offering a deeper process than what is generally possible in a verbal exchange. I also believe that students who had experienced serious difficulties or interruptions in their studies might find that arts-based supervision methods would not be appropriate for them.

The following selected examples of my artwork responses reflect the themes of struggle, challenge and resolution that I derived from the graduate students' comments and artwork about their study experiences over the past year. Some mentioned having to jump through hoops to move forward, to swim through rough water and seek sanctuary and recreation to reflect and restore their energy. My artwork responses echo these themes back to them but also add others that depict the students' insights, growth, strengths and their uses of fulfilling pastimes, such as music and cooking activities, self-care resources for relaxation and nurturance. I also noted the students' aspirations and challenges in the midst of various personal, family and academic challenges. The art and text responses acknowledged the students' efforts and actions during their year of study and also affirmed their struggles and achievements. Below, I include selected art response works and a title that represents what I wanted to convey about the art and narrative provided by the student to me.

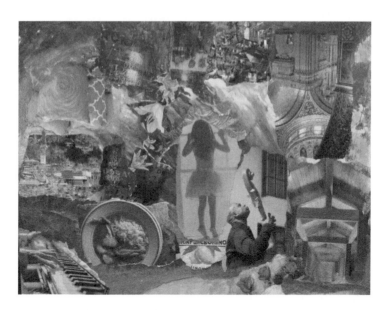

Figure 8.1 Time to finally enjoy life again; no longer looking in from the outside, but actively living after the degree, by Tuula Heinonen.

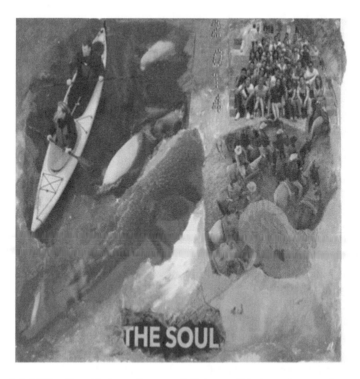

Figure 8.2 With others' help and support, it is possible to overcome dangers and find the way, by Tuula Heinonen.

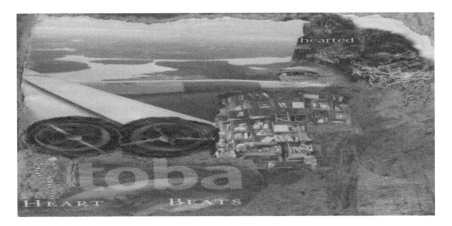

Figure 8.3 Adventurous journeys alongside the demands of study; nurturance and perseverance help, by Tuula Heinonen.

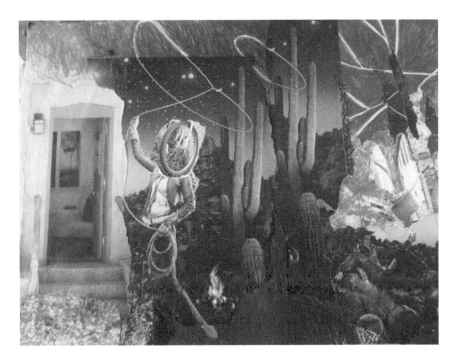

Figure 8.4 Home fires and solid earth; ideas keep turning and spinning; need for grounding, by Tuula Heinonen.

Reflections about the creative exercise

In introducing the art exercise to the graduate students, I wanted to add a creative dimension to an annual review that was usually dominated by standard meeting procedures and forms. I also wanted the exercise to include a reciprocal process in which I would view and respond to students' collage art and how they interpreted it. The images and other material that they used for the collages came from their homes – magazines, newspapers, crayons and ephemera – and each student thoughtfully placed these on a sheet of paper to represent what the past year of studies consisted of and meant to them. When I met with each one to discuss the artwork, I paid careful attention to what they said and/or wrote and, soon after, produced my response for them. The reciprocal process of making art for one another and sharing impressions of the students' achievements and challenges over the year generated in me a greater respect for the complexity in these mature graduate students' lives and how they were able to conduct their academic work, despite their also performing multiple social roles and the multiplicity of tasks these entailed. It was clear that the knowledge from the students' lived experiences grounded their work, helping them to iteratively adapt and synthesise from learning drawn from course readings, assignments, lectures and discussions. Learning is an ongoing and interactive process of taking in new information, discussing it, reflecting on it in light of one's unique experiences, and then assessing its relevance and utility for application in concrete situations (Kolb 1984, Cheung and Delavega 2014). In the context of a reciprocal relationship that includes meaningful reflection and discussion between graduate student and academic supervisor, it can lead to enriched knowledge and personal transformation, not only for students but also for academic supervisors. The inclusion of creative work as a part of my graduate student supervision helped the students to conceptualise and gain insight related to their studies and their views on the world in which they live, work and study, and how these elements shift and change over time. According to Rudolph Arnheim (1969 cited in Simmons and Daley 2013, p. 1), 'the arts are the most powerful means of strengthening the perceptual component without which productive thinking is impossible in any field of endeavour.' It engages right-brain thinking in which problem-solving and synthesis so reside with creativity (Simmons and Daley 2013).

I hoped that through participating in this creative exercise, students would view their work in new ways and glean insights that would contribute to their graduate work. I also wanted to enhance my graduate student supervision practice and skills in an art-making partnership. Nicola Simmons and Shauna Daley (2013), who made use of collage with university educators and graduate students in a research project, found that collage-making helped the participants to 'get unstuck' and 'see with new eyes' (p. 6), which helped them to 'move beyond cognitive blocks, pushing them forward in their thinking and their ability to reflect at a meta-cognitive level' (p. 7).

I had similar feedback from graduate students and found that, soon after the exercise ended, most of the students became more motivated to move forward in their work, particularly if they were at the point of developing their thesis or advanced practice proposals and reports. It is also possible that the act of reviewing the year's work enhanced their productivity.

I responded to each graduate student about what I observed and heard from our communication and meetings together, concentrating on their strong points and the strategies they used to move forward in their studies. In addition, I heard how students had struggled with challenges, such as family and employment responsibilities, time constraints, writer's block and other setbacks, but also drew from their own repertoires of relaxation, renewal and stress reduction methods to deal with multiple roles and tasks at home, in their jobs and in their student lives. All of them said that the arts-based annual review session was valuable, despite the additional time it took to create their art and describe the challenges they faced and dealt with during the year. I also spent additional time with each student who participated in the art exercise so I could learn from them how I could better support their graduate studies work and understand their needs. This information, I knew, would also contribute to my own continuing educational development in student supervision.

In my response art for the students, I focussed on their unique interests and academic processes. Many told me about how they encountered and struggled to overcome a range of stumbling blocks, from time constraints to new challenges in their work and lives. I believed that it was important for me to include what I heard from them in my response art and affirmation of their successes and significant efforts over the year.

Reciprocity in graduate supervision was significantly enhanced through the arts-based exercise. I developed a greater understanding and appreciation of the complexities in the lives of my graduate students and how they prioritised their studies, making sacrifices all the while. The integration into student supervision of visual methods that involve both student and instructor can open new spaces for reflection and dialogue. Reciprocity in this process adds a deeper dimension to the process of graduate student advising (Halse and Bansel 2012). In addition, art-making is often insightful and enjoyable. Commonalities and differences in experience are found, and opportunities for exchanging ideas and knowledge occur in the process, resulting in what is often a rewarding experience for the student and the supervisor.

Limitations, caveats and conclusion

The inclusion of art-making as part of student supervision may require some time for introduction and orientation, and in some cases, it may not be appropriate at all. Regarding supervision for counsellors using play therapy, Patrick Morrissette and Shannon Gadbois (2006) refer to a number of potential problems that can arise in using creative techniques in counselling.

They mention that supervisees may experience discomfort when taking part in these methods as they may bring up personal issues that the supervisors may not want to discuss. The arts can delve into and bring up human experiences that are more easily shielded in verbal exchanges. Another possible drawback is that those being supervised may want to perform well to please their supervisors, who they perceive as having power over their academic progress. Students need to be told about the option of not taking part in creative exercises and given the choice to opt out.

For graduate students who have had negative experiences or criticism regarding their making art or skill in producing art, an arts-based exercise may be unappealing and could be a barrier to reciprocity between the student and an academic supervisor. Such students may prefer discussions with their supervisors over an added component involving art-making and discussion about the artwork. Alternatively, students who have well-developed artistic skill and/or experience may want to focus on executing an aesthetically attractive art product over creating art to focus on reflection and discussion of their studies. Students need to be oriented to the purpose of a creative component in the supervision experience so they determine for themselves if they wish to participate and how they can benefit from it in the supervisory relationship.

If difficult events or transitions have taken place and affected a student's studies or personal life, reflection and art-making may generate distress and/or cause them to relive uncomfortable experiences (Hyun *et al.* 2006). Support is needed for any students who experience adverse emotional reactions, whether as a result of art-making or during discussion in supervision meetings.

Academic supervisors who are not comfortable with arts-based media or creative activities in supervision might find such initiatives challenging or confusing. As a result, they would likely find it difficult to carry out arts-based supervision effectively and facilitate the interpretation of artwork by their students. The creation of artwork in response to the students' art may also not be of interest to some academic supervisors.

Arts-based methods offer creative and interesting complements to more conventional methods used in graduate student supervision. Their use needs to fit with the purposes and context in which the supervision takes place, the skills and interests of the supervisor and the students, and the acceptance of complementary methods and reciprocity in student-academic supervisor relationships. This chapter has described the inclusion of visual art, primarily collage, as an element of graduate supervision, a reciprocal process enhanced by mutual reflection and discussion shaped by creative activity and exchange.

In summary, using an arts-based method in graduate student supervision can be enjoyable, stimulating and interesting for both students and advisors. New ideas and perspectives and enhanced motivation and/or direction might result from integrating creative methods. For students who enjoy reflection through art-making and find it inspiring or enlightening, much can be learned from reciprocal sharing that occurs through creative expression with advisors. For students who prefer only advisor-student meetings, arts-based supervisory alternatives may not be very useful and might even impede the advisor-student relationship. This does not mean that reciprocity in the relationship is limited but that more conventional methods, such as face-to-face meetings, would work better. For such students, traditional methods of supervision are preferable. Arts-based supervisory methods may lead to greater reciprocity in the relationship between graduate students and their advisors but only if students (and advisors) are open to the introduction of creativity and art-making for the purpose of promoting reflexivity and reciprocity.

References

Acker, S., 2011. Reflections on supervision and culture: What difference does difference make? *Innovations in Education and Teaching International*, 48 (4), 413–420.

Barrett, T. and Hussey, J., 2015. Overcoming problems in doctoral writing through the use of visualisations: Telling our stories. *Teaching in Higher Education*, 20 (1), 48–63.

Bernard, J. and Goodyear, R., 2004. *Fundamentals of clinical supervisions* (3rd ed.). Boston, MA: Allyn & Bacon.

Bonnycastle, M. and Bonnycastle, C., 2015. Photographs generate knowledge: Reflections on experiential learning in/outside the social work classroom. *Journal of Teaching in Social Work*, 35 (3), 233–250.

Butler-Kisber, L., 2010. *Qualitative inquiry: Thematic, narrative and arts-informed perspectives*. Thousand Oaks, CA: Sage.

Buunk, B., Doosje, B., Jans, L. and Hopstaken, L., 1993. Perceived reciprocity, social support, and stress at work: The role of exchange and communal orientation. *Journal of Personality and Social Psychology*, 65 (4), 801–811.

Cassidy, S., 2009. Subjectivity and the valid assessment of pre-registration student nurse clinical learning outcomes: Implications for mentors. *Nurse Education Today*, 29 (1), 33–39.

Cheung, M. and Delavega, E., 2014. Five-way experiential learning model for social work education. *Social Work Education: The International Journal*, 33 (8), 1070–1087.

Coholic, D., Lougheed, S. and Lebreton, J., 2009. The helpfulness of holistic arts-based group work with children living in foster care. *Social Work with Groups*, 32 (1–2), 29–46.

Conrad, D. and Sinner, A., eds., 2015. *Creating together: Participatory, community-based, and collaborative arts practices and scholarship across Canada*. Waterloo, ON: Wilfrid Laurier University Press.

Coulshed, V., 1993. Adult learning: Implications for teaching in social work education. *British Journal of Social Work*, 23 (1), 1–13.

Deaver, S. and Shiflett, C., 2011. Art-based supervision techniques. *The Clinical Supervisor* [online], 30 (2), 257–276. doi: 10.1080/07325223.2011.619456.

Desyallas, M. and Sinclair, A., 2014. Zine-making as a pedagogical tool for transformative learning in social work education. *Social Work Education*, 33 (3), 296–316.

Fish, B., 2008. Formative evaluation research of arts-based supervision in art therapy training. *Art Therapy: Journal of the American Art Therapy Association*, 25 (2), 70–77.

Gurr, G., 2001. Negotiating the rackety bridge – A dynamic model for aligning supervisory style with research student development. *Higher Education Research & Development*, 20, 81–82.

Halse, C., 2011. 'Becoming a supervisor': The impact of doctoral supervision on supervisors' learning. *Studies in Higher Education*, 36 (5), 557–570.

Halse, C. and Bansel, P., 2012. The learning alliance: Ethics in doctoral supervision. *Oxford Review of Education*, 38 (4), 377–392.

Harrison, S. and Grant, C., 2015. Exploring new models of research pedagogy: Time to let go of master-apprentice style supervision? *Teaching in Higher Education*, 20 (5), 556–566. doi: 10.1080/13562517.2015.1036732.

Heinonen, T., 2015. *Arts-based expression in social work: Experiences in learning and teaching.* Final project, Vancouver, BC: Vancouver Art Therapy Institute.

Hughes, M., 2012. Unitary appreciative inquiry (UAI): A new approach for re-searching social work education and practice. *British Journal of Social Work*, 42 (7), 1388–1405.

Huss, E., 2012. What we see and what we say: Combining visual and verbal informa-tion within social work research. *British Journal of Social Work*, 42 (8), 1440–1459.

Hyun, J., Quinn, B., Madon, T. and Lustig, S., 2006. Graduate student mental health: Needs assessment and utilization of counseling services. *Journal of College Student Development*, 47 (3), 247–266.

Kalin, N., Barney, D. and Irwin, R., 2009. Complexity thinking mentorship: An emergent pedagogy of graduate research development. *Mentoring and Tutoring: Partnership in Learning*, 17 (4), 10–31.

Keddell, E., 2011. A constructivist approach to the use of arts-based materials in social work education: Making connections between art and life. *Journal of Teaching in Social Work*, 31, 400–414. doi: 10.1080/08841233.2011.597678.

Knowles, M., Holton, E. and Swanson, R., 2015. *The adult learner: The definitive classic in adult education and human resource development.* London: Routledge.

Kolb, D., 1984. *Experiential learning: Experience as the source of learning and devel-opment.* Englewood Cliffs, NJ: Prentice Hall.

Konopik, D. and Cheung, M., 2012. Psychodrama as a social work modality. *Social Work*, 58 (1), 9–20. doi: 1093/sw/sws054.

McArdle, F., Knight, L. and Stratigos, T., 2013. Imagining social justice. *Contempo-rary Issues in Early Childhood*, 14 (4), 357–369.

McAuliffe, G., 2000. How counselor education influences future helpers: What students say. In G. McAuliffe and K. Eriksen (eds.), *Preparing counselors and therapists: Creating constructivist and developmental programs.* Virginia Beach, VA: Donning Publishers for the Association for Counselor Education and Super-vision, 42–61.

Morrissette, P. and Gadbois, S., 2006. Ethical consideration of counselor educa-tion teaching strategies. *Counseling and Values*, 50, 131–141. doi: 10.1002/j.2161–07X.2006.tb00049.x.

Moxley, D., Feen-Callaghan, H. and Washington, O., 2012. Lessons learned from three projects linking social work, the arts, and humanities. *Social Work Educa-tion: The International Journal*, 31 (6), 703–723.

Mulder, C. and Dull, A., 2014. Facilitating self-reflection: The integration of photovoice in graduate social work education. *Social Work Education: The International Journal*, 33 (8), 1017–1036.

Murphy, N., 2009. Research supervision: Matches and mismatches. *International Journal of Electrical Engineering Education*, 46 (3), 295–306.

Newsome, D., Henderson, D. and Veach, L., 2005. Using expressive arts in group supervision to enhance awareness and foster cohesion. *The Journal of Humanistic Counselling, Education and Development*, 44 (2), 145–157.

Shor, I., 1992. *Empowering education: Critical teaching for social change*. Chicago, IL: University of Chicago.

Simmons, N. and Daley, S., 2013. The art of thinking: Using collage to stimulate scholarly work. *Canadian Journal for the Scholarship of Teaching and Learning*, 4 (1), 1–11.

Sinding, C. and Barnes, H., eds., 2015. *Social work artfully: Beyond borders and boundaries*. Waterloo, ON: Wilfrid Laurier University Press.

Vaughan, K., 2003. Pieced together: Collage as an artist's method for interdisciplinary research. *International Journal of Qualitative Methods*, 4 (1), 27–52.

Walton, P., 2012. Beyond talk and text: An expressive visual arts method for social work education. *Social Work Education: The International Journal*, 31 (6), 724–741.

Wehbi, S., 2009. Reclaiming our agency in academia: Engaging in the scholarship of teaching in social work. *Social Work Education*, 28 (5), 502–511.

9 Narrative reflection as a reciprocal interview method

Eveliina Heino and Minna Veistilä

Introduction

In this methodological chapter, we discuss the use of narrative reflection in interview-based research. We aim to describe and analyse elements that render narrative reflection a reciprocal method. Narrative reflection, in this context, refers to presenting, discussing, and interpreting the preliminary results of a study with interviewees. In the literature, many concepts have been used to describe similar approaches to narrative reflection, such as member checking, participant verification, informant feedback, respondent validation, applicability, external validity, and fittingness (Morse *et al.* 2002). Here, we specifically use the concept 'narrative reflection' because, to us, the method not only includes checking our preliminary interpretations but also consists of a narrative approach that creates a shared interpretation with interviewees (Veistilä 2008, see also Frank 2010).

In our study, we focus on reciprocal elements of narrative reflection. Reciprocity is a broad concept that describes an important aspect of social life and intersubjective relations in which all parties experience a gain from one another (see Törrönen and Heino 2013). Intersubjective reciprocity can be viewed as a consequence of acknowledgment, consideration, and self-regulation, that is, learned moral behaviour, that passes from generation to generation (Neusner and Chilton 2008, p. 2, pp. 170–171). It is also possible to approach reciprocity as a virtue based on the notion that good should be returned, bad should be opposed and not returned, and bad notions require compensation. In this way, reciprocity represents an important part of morality and a force uniting societies. However, acts of reciprocity need not be similar. and returning reciprocal acts can take much time (Becker 1990, p. 73).

Despite representing a broad concept that includes multiple aspects, we define reciprocity, using the definition of Antti Kujala and Mirkka Danielsbacka (2015, p. 21), as *an exchange or a system in which all parties experience being treated fairly.* In this research, reciprocity is limited to the interview context. In our analysis, we rely on data from our own studies and scrutinise reciprocity as a part of narrative reflection on a micro level, using concrete examples from our data. In the sections that follow, we first describe narrative reflection in detail and then concentrate on the implementation of our research, our research questions, and the results of our study.

Narrative reflection in social work research

Narratives represent socially constructed human experiences (Ricoeur 1984). In keeping with Jerome Bruner (1987, 1996, p. 123), we understand narratives as both thoughts and stories told. Thus, life can be described and interpreted using narratives, and narratives can represent spoken descriptions of life events. Using narratives allows a researcher to scrutinise the multilayered landscapes of actions and meanings among individuals and families (Squire *et al.* 2013). While individuals produce narratives, those narratives are not created in a vacuum but in relation to, for example, societally recognised reflections about expected actions in certain situations and the values promoted within specific contexts. Thus, humans create narratives in certain contexts using the tools and concepts available to them (Hänninen 2000, pp. 94–143).

As such, 'reflection' as a concept can be transcribed as 'wondering.' In the field of social work, reflection has been used as a method for developing practice. Thus, a social worker can describe her/his feelings and thoughts and reconsider her/his choices. We must also point out that these reflections stand as narratives, that is, they represent the social worker's stories of the way s/he works and thus create a picture of the professional. Carolyn Taylor (2006, p. 194) argues that professional social workers create their own professional identity by analysing narrative reflections from their work. Jaakko Seikkula (1999, pp. 86, 91) defines reflectivity as a process of internal speech transformed into external speech. As such, reality is constructed between the participants of the discussion in a space that allows for a shared understanding when assisted by the active use of language.

In the 21st century, the expertise and knowledge of service-users have been highlighted in social work practice, resulting in the concept of *expertise by experience* This concept relies on the notion that service-users carry personal experiences of certain difficult life situations, and based on these experiences, they participate in developing social work practices (Hyväri and Salo 2009). Expertise by experience has also proved valuable in participatory research. Furthermore, narrative reflection has many links to participatory research, which aims to implement research in partnership with the individuals under study, viewing them as partners in the knowledge production process (Bergold and Thomas 2012; Russo 2012). This form of research includes both planning and conducting research with experts by experience (Törrönen and Vornanen 2014). In general, participatory research is designed to support those with less power and targets the production of democratic knowledge (Hall 2001, p. 171). According to Tina Cook

(2012), participatory research can impact participants, researchers, research design, knowledge about practice, and policy and practice itself.

Regardless of the increased interest in service-users' knowledge of the field of social work and their participation in research, narrative reflection is not a widely used method in social work research. In our research, we applied narrative reflection for several reasons. First, it limits the possibility of mis- or over-interpretation (Creswell 2007). Narrative reflection may also carry a positive therapeutic influence because reading others' interpretations of one's own life situations may increase self-knowledge, enable self-reflection, and produce feelings of being heard (see, for example, Colbourne and Sque 2005, p. 551). Thus, establishing an egalitarian discussion, in which multiple voices are simultaneously heard, represented the ideal for our interviews and analysis, ultimately leading to our choice of narrative reflection as a research method.

We acknowledge that this method does not remove all power structures between the interviewer and interviewees and that it carries certain limitations. Interviews can be described as institutional situations because both the interviewer and interviewees maintain certain roles, and the situation is guided by the goals of the research (Ruusuvuori and Tiittula 2005, p. 23). For example, interviewees may remain polite or trust an expert's opinion, not questioning the interpretations of the researcher. In a worst-case scenario, researchers may pressure interviewees to agree with their interpretations, which can result in the exploitation of the interviewees and cannot be considered as a reciprocal act.

It is also possible that, while reading their life story, repressed memories or feelings will surface and affect the interviewee in various ways. Naturally, shared interpretations may also result in powerful feelings within the researcher and influence her/his thinking and actions (Lowes and Gill 2006). As the authors and qualified social workers, we considered such issues when designing our study. For example, during the interviews, we did not pressure interviewees to reveal any details they did not wish to, showed empathy towards their stories, and did not strictly follow our interview guide if interviewees wanted to talk more about some issues or themes.

Implementation of the research

We collected our research data in 2012 and 2013, when we were both working on the 'Empowerment of Families with Children' project.[1] In this project, we conducted research among families with a Russian background living in South-Eastern Finland. Our doctoral dissertation research focussed on the integration-related construction of well-being and the basic service experiences of families. We requested a random sample of 1,000 individuals' postal addresses from the Finnish Population Register Centre and sent a separate form along with a questionnaire in which we asked if the recipients would be willing to participate in an interview. In total, we reached

25 families willing to participate and interviewed them during the summer of 2012. Based on the preferences of the interviewees, ten interviews were conducted in Russian, eight in Finnish, six in both Finnish and Russian, and one in Russian and English. During 13 interviews, more than one family member was present, such as the interviewee's children and spouse. During 12 interviews, only the migrant family member was present. In addition, during three interviews, grandparents were present, while during two interviews, a family friend was present.

After the first 25 interviews, we selected nine of these families to participate in narrative reflection. These families were interviewed a second time during the summer of 2013. Our selection criteria for the second interview consisted of representativeness of the families. Thus, we chose families representing differing ages, varying reasons for receiving residence permits, various locations, and varying lengths of time having lived in Finland. The interviews lasted from 30 minutes to 2.5 hours. These two sets of interviews lasted a total of 53.5 hours, amounting to 416 pages of transcribed data.

After the first interview, we drafted our interpretations of the narratives from nine families in the form of one-page summaries. We wrote these narratives from the different points of view that emerged during the interviews. The heading for each narrative was 'x family's experiences of well-being and the service system.' The interviewed families read our interpretations in Finnish or Russian. We then discussed the summaries, recording what the family members had to say about our interpretations.

The data from this study has been used in several publications (e.g. Heino 2016, Veistilä 2016). This chapter, however, focusses on the methodological aspects of our data collection. Thus, our research question here is '*What are the reciprocal elements of narrative reflection?*'

We focus on the structure of the interviews and the different ways in which we interacted during the interview processes. Upon a closer examination of narrative reflection, we clarify the manifold meanings of reciprocity within the research interview process. We use content analysis as an analytical tool, and interview excerpts illustrate reciprocal elements in our interpretations of the data. We take reciprocal elements to mean *the parts of narrative reflection that promote reciprocity between the researchers and the interviewees*. Our analysis proceeded with a detailed reading of the data and a thematic division of fragments of text, which formed a part of the narrative reflection. Next, we grouped together fragments describing reciprocity. These fragments were divided into three sub-themes: creating shared interpretations, participation, and recognition, which we call the *reciprocal elements of narrative reflection*. The final, more in-depth stage of analysis involved an exploration of these three elements in greater detail. Throughout this chapter, the names of the interviewees have been changed to preserve their anonymity. Interviewees' names used in the interview excerpts are pseudonyms.

Elements that promote reciprocity

Creating shared interpretations

Creating shared interpretations of events and discussions between researchers and interviewees emerged as the first element of narrative reflection that
we identified. Part of this element consisted of validating biographical details, for instance, when we erroneously recorded details during an interview,
such as a relative's name or a child's age. When we met with the interviewees
the second time, they corrected us. In many cases, however, we started an
entirely new discussion or were able to discuss previously reviewed topics in
greater detail. In this way, *presenting the interviewees* became an important
part of the discussion during the second interviews:

EVELIINA: We wrote up your story – that is, our interpretation of it. We
would like to ask you to read it and comment on it. Is there something
we need to add or correct?

STANISLAV: Well, I would like to correct this part: 'I do not know how I will
manage to pay our bills and the loan.' I do know how to manage this. It
is difficult, but not impossible. We pay everything, but our standard of
living has fallen. We are living on the edge; we do have food, but because
there is less money, things are more difficult.

MINNA: This is exactly why it is so important to talk with you again, so that
no misunderstandings remain.

STANISLAV: This part: 'When I moved to Finland, I did not know what to do
and how to be.' I knew what to do, because I came here to work. But how
to be… do nothing wrong, and everything will be well. I was looking a
bit… the culture is so different here. It is different when just visiting here
and then returning to one's own country. But when you live in this community, you have to understand what is allowed and what is not, the fine
details. At first, I lived very carefully and looked around, looked at how
the other people behaved. In principle, everything is similar – if you do
nothing wrong, you experience no problems.

The narratives we wrote based on the initial interviews were only one page
long. This example illustrates how some important aspects were missing or
how our interpretation seemed too straightforward and somehow presented
the interviewee's situation too simplistically. Regardless of the research
project, the ways in which interviewees are represented remain relevant,
particularly in research among minorities and migrants. Thus, researchers
need to thoroughly ensure that their interpretations avoid promoting oth-
erness (Martikainen 2009, p. 7). In this case, narrative reflection enabled
a discussion about the representations of the interviewees as individuals
and as a group. It also allowed us to consider the structural framework of
Finnish society and to highlight this clearly in our interpretations. In this

way, the challenges that migrant families face do not seem to arise only from themselves nor solely from their cultural backgrounds (also Malkki 1995, Ikäläinen *et al.* 2003). Thus, the discussions that took place during the second interviews allowed us to reflect upon our interpretations and understanding of the phenomena under our study.

The second important aspect of creating a shared understanding consisted of *checking how issues are represented.* For example, during the initial interviews, we explained to the interviewees that we would protect their anonymity in our research. Yet during narrative reflection, questions about anonymity arose:

EVELIINA: After we met, we wrote our interpretation of what you shared with us. We have written this in both Finnish and Russian from your daughter's point of view. We would like you all to read it, and if necessary correct it or comment on it.

MINNA: After we met, we got the feeling that the child's and young people's voices must be heard more, which is why we wrote the summary from her point of view. Then, we wondered if we had understood your story in the right way at all.

EVELIINA: We will not publish the summary as it is here, and your names will not appear with it; we just wanted to make sure...

ARTEM: There was, in my narrative, but I was nervous [...] I spoke too much about myself.

MINNA: ...but that is why we are here, so that we can change the details if you feel we need to, and because we understand that situations do change.

MARIA: Everything is true except [the bit about] the gifts. I am the kind of a person who likes to give presents.

ARTEM: It is true. But the critique against Russia, you have to remove our names. Do you know the situation? Well, it is a bit dangerous.

MINNA: Yes, of course. We will remove your names, and we can also change your ages and occupations so that you cannot be recognised.

EVELIINA: And, we are interested in phenomena at a general level. We do not normally focus on one specific family for our research nor report that you specifically said this. We will not publish summaries like this; we try to write about general experiences about well-being and services.

In this example, the family interviewed expressed concern regarding our interpretation of their situation, an interpretation that seemed too bold to them. They were also concerned about their anonymity. During the second interview, we were able to discuss and reflect upon these issues with them, issues that proved worrisome to the interviewees. At times, protecting the anonymity of interviewees competes with presenting research data to support researchers' interpretations (for example, see Josselson 2007, pp. 541–542). We found, however, that a shared understanding overcame this competition, that is, ensured the interviewees' anonymity by removing information, such as their home cities, and by changing their names, ages, and professions.

Reciprocity as fairness served as an element in creating shared interpretations of the results with interviewees. Furthermore, interviewees had an opportunity to reflect upon their own life stories, and we were able to reflect upon our interpretations and understandings of the results as well as the ethical issues related to our research.

Participation

Contemporary social work theories stress the importance of participation from ethical and legal points of view (see, for example, Payne 2014). Harry Shier (2006, p. 17) defines the participation of children in a way that suits interviewee participation in the analysis of research quite well. According to his theory of pathways to participation, three dimensions and five stages of participation exist. The dimensions consist of *openings, obligations,* and *opportunities.* As such, openings focus on individual readiness to act; obligations focus on the resources, tools, and methods available to individuals; and opportunities refer to the political and legal possibilities open to individuals (Shier 2006, p. 19).

Furthermore, Shier (2006) defined five stages of participation. During the first stage, a person must be *listened to.* In interview research, this means that the interviewer must be ready to listen to what the interviewee has to say without bringing her/his own assumptions or opinions to the discussion. The interviewer must possess the capacity to listen, and contemporary research policy must support listening to the interviewees. In most contemporary interview research, this is the case. During the second stage of participation, individuals must be *supported to express their views.* Current interview techniques and research policies primarily support this stage as well.

During the third stage, the interviewees' *views must be taken into account.* This is where narrative reflection comes into play. Not only did we listen to the interviewees, but our choice of method allowed us to support their influence on our research findings and conclusions. Here, participation refers not only to the interviewees' active role in the interview process but also to their role in the analysis. Narrative reflection afforded interviewees the possibility of participating in the detailed analysis of well-being and service experiences. This included the defining of central concepts:

MINNA: We have identified these different concepts regarding the process: adaptation, integration, and assimilation. What do you think we should talk about?

VENERA: To my mind, first, adaptation and, then, integration. I think there are two stages. First, adaptation. In a way, this includes the first steps – getting to know the environment and people around you, all the things here and adapting to being and behaving the way people do here. Integration starts when you know these and create your own life according to it. When you have the networks, friends, services, working life, and daily routines, then you in a way come home. I think that you first adapt and then integrate...

MINNA: Are there different stages in different families?

VENERA: Most likely there are, and from these first steps it depends on what kinds of people you happen to meet along the way.

Here, we see that the interviewer was interested in the different concepts that emerged during the initial interview. She asked the interviewee an open question: 'What do you think we should talk about?' Instead of choosing one, the interviewee wanted to bring up a new idea, which included two different stages. The interviewer accepted the idea and took it further by asking if the stages differed within different families. Again, the interviewee was able to describe a new angle to the concept by addressing how these stages differed because of migrant families' multiple relationships. In this way, the interviewee meaningfully participated by defining the research concepts.

Participation as a reciprocal element of narrative reflection also included using the interviewees' expertise by further developing shared interests:

MINNA: I am still thinking about the bullying of your son at school. How do you think these kinds of things should be addressed so that they do not happen again?

JOSEFINA: As a mother, I would send a psychologist and a social worker to those boys' families. I would let them work on the situation. Nowadays, children have become very cruel, and it is because of the families – that is, the things that happen within families.

MINNA: That sounds good. Nowadays, I think that what they do is move the bullied child into another class, which does not solve anything in itself.

Here, the interviewee was asked to solve a problem for which she had a clear solution, which the interviewer validated by saying, 'That sounds good' and providing an example of another, less desirable solution to the problem. This allowed the interviewee to expand upon her thinking about how families act and the reasons for such actions in a detailed manner. Furthermore, this allows the interviewee to participate in reflecting on an important societal problem.

The fourth and fifth stages of the pathways to participation challenge researchers to *involve the interviewees in decision-making processes* and allow them to *share responsibility and decision-making power* (Shier 2006, p. 17). We have not yet reached these stages, wherein interviewees serve as co-authors on interviewers' publications. As younger scholars, we are not yet brave enough to challenge conventional dissertation practices and policies.

However, this represents an interesting reciprocal possibility that we plan to continue moving towards in our future research.

Recognition

The concept of recognition is usually understood as containing at least the subjective and intersubjective poles. The subjective pole is described using attributes such as love, respect, and appreciation, that is, attitudes. But attitude alone is insufficient because of the demand for intersubjectivity. This means that recognition must be expressed in such a way that another person understands and accepts this attitude (Honneth 2001, p. 115, Ikäheimo 2003, pp. 127–128). Thus, in our analysis, recognition consists of being heard, reflection, and a shared appreciation of the research itself.

Hearing the opinions of service users can be seen as necessary and as an important component of social work practice. Typically, during research interviews, the researcher asks the interviewees some questions, the interviewees answer these questions, and then the researcher may ask some additional questions and summarise the discussion. Depending upon the situation, this type of interview does not necessarily allow interviewees to feel that they are heard because the researcher makes her/his own interpretations about the interview afterwards without consulting the participants.

When applying narrative reflection, the setting differs from the institutional practice of interviewing because interviewees are provided the opportunity to comment on the researchers' interpretations of participant narratives and what these expressed. In our research, this was accomplished by allowing our interviewees to read our interpretations of the initial interviews, affording them the experience of *being heard:*

MINNA: This (story) will not be published; we had an idea for this kind of story when we heard it. We thought of writing it from the perspective of a young girl who was writing a diary.

VENERA: It is just like this! It is just like this! It is really just like this! Oh my, it is like this. It is about a breakthrough after graduation, when I started to find friends and about that difficult time and about my friend who was important and about the present time, about our family. Really, it is just so right.

MINNA: It's nice to hear this. This story was so touching that we wanted to write it in that way as well. But, we were also wondering what could have helped in that kind of a situation? What services could somehow be useful?

In this example, the interviewee was surprised and impressed after reading our interpretation of her narrative. She explained her reaction, stating that participation in this research was the only situation in which it was possible for her to recall and retell the entire story related to her migration and integration. She expressed having an experience of being heard during the first interview. But according to her telling, the second interview and subsequent reading of our interpretation helped her to understand and make sense of her own experiences.

After discussing the story and her feelings related to it, we could discuss the practical implications for basic services aimed at supporting migrants. Viewing the interviewees' opinions as expert opinions diminishes the power differential between the researcher and the interviewees. In general, most interviewees expressed their joy when they felt that their stories were valued and welcomed, given that we used our time with them to discuss those experiences.

The second part of recognition is *reflection*, which consists of the possibility of self-reflection and reflection on the phenomenon in general, along with reflection on one's own experiences as a part of that phenomenon (see also Bergold and Thomas 2012). Reading the narratives from their own lives enabled the interviewees to self-reflect on their life events and the choices they made:

STANISLAV: I thought more about being a driver. Many people have asked me why I did not go to study, why I went straight to work. I haven't thought about it much and probably only started thinking about it a few years ago. I understood that it is for my family. I have a family; I have to feed my family – my small child, wife... I do not have time for studies. When I read this story, I thought about this once again. And here I am working, making money. And being a driver was my dream.

Many interviewees mentioned that the topics discussed during the interviews were issues that they had not thought about in a long while. Thus, narrative reflection enabled self-reflection and functioned as recognition because it made our interpretations visible. Thus, reading their own stories made it possible for the interviewees *to reflect upon broader phenomena* impacting them in general, such as migration and integration:

MINNA: Some of our interviewees described the process of moving to another country as one where you must forget your previous self and re-construct yourself from the beginning; after that re-construction is complete, you can then look backwards.

VENERA: It is possible to compare yourselves at some point. That is true. In my case, it was a good thing that I was so young. So I was taking care of things almost as any young Finnish person would. But there were a few more difficulties.

Recognition in these interviews also included recognition of the meaning of migration, the demand for integration, and feelings related to these processes. The third area of recognition centred around the interviewees and researchers' expressing a *shared appreciation of the research*. In this way, the researchers and their work were also acknowledged by the interviewees:

MINNA: If you had some person coming to you who could promote your well-being in these services, who would that be?
VIKTOR: Aren't we doing that right now?
MINNA: We hope so.
VIKTOR: I want to clarify that I trust the research. [...] Because, if there is no research, there is no development; if there is no such thing, the wheels will stop. So those things go hand in hand.

A shared appreciation of the research can be interpreted as reciprocal recognition because the researchers recognised the importance of the issues that the interviewees experienced, and the interviewees recognised the importance of the study conducted by the researchers. In this way, recognition was reciprocal.

Conclusions

This chapter aims to identify the reciprocal elements of narrative reflection. In our analysis, we focussed on the structure of the interviews and the different ways of interacting with participants during the interview process. We define reciprocal elements as those parts of narrative reflection that promote reciprocity between the researchers and the interviewees. These elements consisted of creating shared interpretations, participation, and recognition. Through these elements, reciprocity as experiencing fairness (Kujala and Danielsbacka 2015) was promoted in three ways. First, the interviewees had a chance to reflect upon narratives constructed by us, while we had the chance to reflect upon our interpretations and understandings of the results as well as the ethical issues of our research. The interviewees recounted that reading our interpretations of the initial interviews allowed them to feel heard because it was possible for them to remember and retell their stories of migration and integration during the interviews. This proved helpful in understanding and interpreting their own experiences.

Second, discussions during the second interviews allowed for reflection upon our interpretations and an understanding of the phenomena under study. Here, we consulted and created a shared understanding of the results with the interviewees. Furthermore, interviewees had the opportunity to influence the research findings. Finally, the interviewees expressed their appreciation of this research. In this way, the interviewees acknowledged the researchers as well as their work.

Our primary research question in this chapter focussed on the reciprocal elements of narrative reflection. Yet we should also recognise the limitations and tensions that render the method non-reciprocal. One limitation is that narrative reflection, like any participatory research, requires a safe space and a democratic society. Otherwise, it may not be possible for interviewees to freely express critical opinions. Furthermore, differential ethical and power issues related to this method, such as how interviewees are chosen, whose voices are heard, who decides what issues are discussed, who controls the research, and who benefits from it, invite further discussion (Bergold and Thomas 2012).

According to Atkinson (2001, p. 133), in narrative research, the interaction and relationship between the researcher and the interviewee greatly affect the form and content of the narratives that the researcher receives. We found an emotional aspect strongly present in our interviews, indicating just how important it is for the researcher to gain the trust of interviewees. In our experience, trust was easily obtained during the second interview because both parties were familiar with one another, knew what to expect, and could express themselves more openly. In a traditional research setting, the interview is institutionalised, and the researcher and interviewee assume particular roles (Ruusuvuori 2010, p. 269). By using narrative reflection, we found it possible to alter these roles and provide greater opportunities for the interviewees to bring their own expertise in the discussion.

In conclusion, we found that using narrative reflection is possible in different fields of qualitative research because of the method's constructionist nature. Yet we understand that the goal of research is rarely to create a shared understanding of interpretations or a consensus among researchers and interviewees. Rather, research often seeks to describe, understand, and analyse different phenomena. In contexts in which researchers' and interviewees' values or interests completely diverge, narrative reflection still allows for the close scrutiny of interviewee narratives. During the second interview, researchers may ask more detailed questions than during initial interviews and may search for similarities and differences between interviews. In our research, we completed follow-up interviews and discussed our interpretations with interviewees only once. In turn, interviewees commented and corrected our interpretations on a general level, although not in manuscripts submitted as journal articles. In the future, we hope to take narrative reflection one step further and plan to discuss our interpretations with the interviewees during the later stages of our research as well.

Note

1 This project was implemented from 2011 to 2014 and was coordinated by the University of Helsinki's Palmenia Center for Continuing Education within the Kotka Unit.

References

Atkinson, R., 2001. The Life Story Interview. *In:* J.F. Gubrium and J.A. Holstein, eds. *Handbook of Interview Research. Context and Method.* California: Sage, 121–140.

Becker, L.C., 1990. *Reciprocity.* London: Routledge and Kegan Paul.

Bergold, J., and Thomas, S. 2012. Participatory research methods: A methodological approach in motion. *Historical Social Research*, 37(4), 191–222.

Bruner, J., 1987. Life as a narrative. *Social Research*, 54 (1), 11–32.

Bruner, J., 1996. *The Culture of Education*. Cambridge: Harvard University Press.

Colbourne, L., and Sque, M., 2005. The culture of cancer and the therapeutic impact of qualitative research interviews. *Journal of Research in Nursing*, 10 (5), 551–567.

Cook, T., 2012. Where participatory approaches meet pragmatism in funded (health) research: The challenge of finding meaningful spaces. *Forum: Qualitative Social Research*, 13 (1), Art. 18. Available from: http://nbn-resolving.de/urn:nbn:de:0114-fqs1201187 [Accessed 8 June 2017].

Creswell, J.W., 2007. *Qualitative inquiry and research design: Choosing among five traditions*. 2nd ed. California: Sage.

Finnish Constitution 731/1999.

Frank, A.W., 2010. *Letting Stories Breathe. A Socio-narratology*. Chicago and London: The University of Chicago Press.

Hall, B.L., 2001. I wish this were a poem of practices of participatory research. *Handbook of action research. Participative inquiry and practice*. London: Sage, 171–178.

Heino, E., 2016. Ymmärrystä ja tukea – kohtaamattomuutta ja vääryyttä. Venäläistaustaisten perheiden institutionaalisen luottamuksen ja epäluottamuksen rakentuminen suomalaisia peruspalveluita kohtaan. *Yhteiskuntapolitiikka*, 81 (2), 127–137.

Honneth, A., 2001. Invisibility: On the epistemology of "recognition". *The Aristotelian Society Supplementary*, 75 (1), 111–126.

Hyväri, S., and Salo, M., 2009. *Elämäntarinoista kokemustutkimukseen*. Helsinki: Mielenterveyden keskusliitto.

Hänninen, V., 2000. *Sisäinen tarina, elämä ja muutos*. Tampere: Tampereen yliopisto.

Ikäheimo, H., 2003. Tunnustus, subjektiviteetti ja inhimillinen elämänmuoto. Tutkimuksia Hegelistä ja persoonien välisistä tunnustussuhteista. Thesis (PhD). University of Jyväskylä.

Ikäläinen, S., Martiskainen, T., and Törrönen, M., 2003. *Mangopuun juurelta kuusen katveeseen*. Helsinki: Lastensuojelun keskusliitto.

Josselson, R., 2007. Narrative research and the challenge of accumulating knowledge. *Narrative Inquiry*, 16 (1), 3–10.

Kujala, A., and Danielsbacka, M., 2015. Johdanto: Vallanpitäjien ja kansan keskinäiset velvollisuudet. *In:* A. Kujala and M. Danielsbacka, eds. *Hyvinvointivaltion loppu? Vallanpitäjät, kansa ja vastavuoroisuus*. Helsinki: Tammi, 11–23.

Lowes, L., and Gill, P., 2006. Participants' experiences of being interviewed about an emotive topic. *Journal of Advanced Nursing*, 55 (5), 587–595.

Malkki, L., 1995. *Purity and Exile: Violence, Memory, and National Cosmology among Hutu Refugees in Tanzania*. Thesis (PhD). University of Chicago

Martikainen, T., 2009. Eettisiä kysymyksiä maahanmuuttotutkimuksessa. *Elore, Suomen Kansantietouden Tutkijain Seura ry*, 16 (2), 1–7.

Morse, J. *et al.*, 2002. Verification strategies for establishing reliability and validity in qualitative research. *International Journal of Qualitative Methods*, 1 (2), 1–19.

Neusner, J., and Chilton, B.D., 2008. *The Golden Rule. The Ethics of Reciprocity in World Religions*. Great Britain: Cromwell Press Ltd.

Payne, M., 2014. *Modern Social Work Theory*. London: Palgrave Macmillan.

Ricoeur, P., 1984. *Time and Narrative, Volume 1*. Chicago: The University of Chicago Press.

Russo, J., 2012. Survivor-controlled research: A new foundation for thinking about psychiatry and mental health. *Forum: Qualitative Social Research*, 13 (1), Art. 8.

Available from: http://www.qualitative-research.net/index.php/fqs/article/view/ 1790 [Accessed 8 June 2017].

Ruusuvuori, J., 2010. Vuorovaikutus ja valta haastattelussa – Keskusteluanalyyttinen näkökulma. *In*: J. Ruusuvuori, P. Nikander and M. Hyvärinen, eds. *Hastattelun analyysi.* Tampere: Vastapaino.

Ruusuvuori, J., and Tiittula, L., 2005. Tutkimushaastattelu ja vuorovaikutus. *In:* J. Ruusuvuori and L. Tiittula, eds. *Haastattelu. Tutkimus, tilanteet ja vuorovaikutus.* Tampere: Vastapaino, 22–56.

Seikkula, J., 1999. Reflektiivinen tiimi ja avoin dialogi - kun itse keskustelu tulee tärkeimmäksi. *In:* J. Aaltonen and R. Rinne, eds. *Perhe terapiassa. Vuoropuhelua vuosituhannen vaihtuessa.* Jyväskylä: Suomen Mielenterveysseuran Koulutuskeskus, 84–94.

Shier, H., 2006. *Pathways to Participation Revisited: Nicaragua Perspective.* Available from: http://www.harryshier.net/docs/Shier-Pathways_to_Participation_Revisited_ NZ2006.pdf [Accessed 9 January 2016].

Squire, C., Andrews, M., and Tamboukou, M., 2013. Introduction: What is narrative research? *In:* M. Andrews, C. Squire and M. Tamboukou, eds. *Doing Narrative Research.* London: Sage Publications Ltd.

Taylor, C., 2006. Narrating significant experience: Reflective accounts and the production of (self) knowledge. *British Journal of Social Work*, 36, 189–206.

Törrönen, M., and Heino, E., 2013. Vastavuoroisuus sosiaalityössä. *In*: E. Heino, M. Veistilä, P. Hännikkäinen, T. Vauhkonen, and N. Kärmeniemi, eds. *Vastavuoroiset ja voimaantumista tukevat käytännöt perhetyön kehittämisessä.* Kotka: Koulutus- ja kehittämiskeskus Palmenia, 15–20.

Törrönen, M., and Vornanen, R., 2014. Young people leaving care: Participatory research to improve child welfare practices and the rights of children and young people. *Australian Social Work*, 67 (1), 135–150.

Veistilä, M., 2008. *Päihteitä käyttäneet äidit, heidän lapsensa ja lastensuojelu. Kertomuksia ja reflektioita.* Julkaisuja 2. Lahti: Päijät-Hämeen ja Itä-Uudenmaan sosiaalialan osaamiskeskus Verso.

Veistilä, M., 2016. *Muutosta hyvinvointiin. Tutkimus venäläistaustaisten lapsiperheiden sosiaalisen hyvinvoinnin rakentamisesta integraatioprosesseissa.* Kymenlaakson ammattikorkeakoulun julkaisuja. Sarja A. Nro 75.

10 Negotiating the research space between young people and adults in a PAR study exploring school bullying

Niamh O'Brien, Tina Moules and Carol Munn-Giddings

Introduction

This chapter will focus on the active involvement of five young researchers and an adult researcher in a Participatory Action Research (PAR) project exploring bullying in their school. The study was conducted in the secondary school of an independent day and boarding school in the East of England. Over the course of the research, a reciprocal relationship developed between the young researchers and an adult researcher (first author). Issues of power and recognising each other's unique contributions to the process were features of this reciprocal relationship. The young researchers were self-selected from educational year eight (age 12) to year ten (age 14), and they called themselves *Research for You (R4U)* with the caption, *'Researching for Life without Fear'*. These young researchers and the first author formed the research team. The young researchers were involved with the first author in the development of research methods aimed towards the whole school, including parents and teachers; in co-analysing the data and in presenting and disseminating the findings.

During the study, the participatory process was evaluated on three occasions. Each evaluation fed into the next to provide an in-depth appraisal of how participation happened and the relationships that developed as a result. This chapter will explore and critique these evaluations. Findings from the study are discussed elsewhere (O'Brien *et al.* forthcoming). The chapter will begin by exploring the literature on developing relationships with children and young people through the research process.

Developing relationships with children and young people through the research process

In a traditional research context, the adult holds the power as the 'expert' on what to research about children and young people, how data is collected and, indeed, how data is interpreted (Woodhead and Faulkner 2008). Childhood research, therefore, has traditionally been framed around professional, policy or academic agendas but rarely from the agenda of the child. However, this viewpoint is shifting, and more recently, children have been regarded as active researchers conducting their own research into areas relevant to their everyday lives, sometimes as sole researchers (see Kellett *et al.* 2004) or co-researchers (see Stoudt 2009) and even as commissioners of research (see O'Brien and Moules 2013). This shift recognises children as individuals alongside adults, not separate from them. If opportunities for children to be involved in knowledge production rather than recipients of adult-generated knowledge are provided, children can enable adults to theorise and understand the social world that they occupy (James 2007).

This progressed relationship is certainly not without its limitations, and adult researchers need to be transparent about how issues of power between adult and child researchers are explored and understood in the research project (James 2007, Mannion 2009). It has been suggested that one way to redress these power imbalances is for adults and children to negotiate the research space together through 'intergenerational and interpersonal dialogues' (Mannion 2009, p. 338). Sara Bragg and Michael Fielding (2005) suggest in their educational research that if the involvement of students as researchers is to be productive and engaging, systems need to be put in place to enable dialogue and allow adults and children to listen to and learn from each other. The authors suggest that this is more than collaboration – it is about collegiality and changing our understanding of what it is to be a teacher and what it is to be a student. For the children and adults involved, the relationship becomes interdependent and can begin to flourish as they strive to understand and appreciate each other's unique roles (Fielding 2004, Mannion 2009). In their study involving young people as co-researchers, Niamh O'Brien and Tina Moules (2007) found that using cycles of action and reflection at all stages of the project, even in an informal manner, enabled the research team to challenge some underlying power issues between adults and children. Consequently, changes were made as the project progressed, and the young researchers participated in decision-making alongside adults.

Although there is an emphasis on collaborating with children on their terms, Mary Kellett (2010) advocates that listening to the views of children is not the same as involving them in the decision-making process. Greg Mannion (2007) proposes that involving children in decision-making and actively hearing their voices is useful as a starting point. However, traditionally, adults have made decisions about research without input from children. Rachael Fox (2013) discusses how academic institutions are not usually aware of how children can actively participate in research, and constraints are in place, making their participation difficult. Mannion (2007, 2009) and Kellett (2010) propose that listening is dependent on adults' relinquishing some of the control and power over decisions made during the research and suggest that if this is not realised, then children are relying on adults to facilitate their views. Certainly, children have criticised adults for not providing them with feedback about how their opinions influenced decisions (Davey

2010). Fielding (2004) further stipulates that if students are only asked to participate in consultations and/or research where the agenda and questions have been set by teachers using language that they cannot relate to or the results of which do not relate to them, it is likely that they will feel alienated and patronised and therefore not want to participate in the research. 'Students and teachers need each other, need to work as active partners in the process if it is to be either worthwhile or successful' (Fielding 2004, p. 307).

Accordingly, children need to be invited to join the dialogue with adults and to negotiate how they would like to be involved and how adults can facilitate their participation (Fitzgerald *et al.* 2009, Mannion 2009). Barry Percy-Smith (2015) recognises that participation is more about the process of democracy in which people work together to make decisions and influence change rather than always about having a say. In essence, the quality of the relationships between adults and children and how they actively collaborate is the main component of children's participation (Fielding 2004, Percy-Smith 2015).

Evaluating children's participation in research

For research dedicated to hearing children's voices to be successful, researchers need to use appropriate techniques that do not exclude or patronise children (Kellett *et al.* 2004). Rachel Hinton (2008) suggests that UK researchers are particularly concerned with issues of reliability and the validity of data collected by and from children. In the case of qualitative research, this quality is assessed through the 'trustworthiness' of the research. One way to ensure that child-conducted research is truly child-centred and focussed on what children are telling adults from their perspective is through the evaluation of the process. This, in turn, adds to the trustworthiness of the study. Evaluating children's participation is not about testing to see if it was done correctly or if milestones were reached but more about critically reflecting on the process and learning from it (Percy-Smith and Malone 2001, Sinclair 2004, Davey 2010). In this way, children's participation becomes achievable (Percy-Smith and Malone 2001).

PAR and hearing children's voices

Participatory methodologies have been particularly appropriate for the study of childhood, and PAR has proven popular in ascertaining children's views and involving them directly in the research process. Claire O'Kane (2008, p. 151) suggests that social researchers can: '...play an important role in embracing the challenge to create space for children and young people to be listened to and heard, and I would advocate that the use of participatory techniques would facilitate such a task.'

The process of participatory research makes this methodology successful with children and includes a commitment to continuous information sharing, reflection and action (Winter and Munn-Giddings 2001, O'Kane 2008).

This current study followed three PAR cycles, each involving a process of planning, acting, observing and reflecting, resulting in a revised plan of action as observed by Stephen Kemmis and Robin McTaggart (1988). Each cycle fed into the next. Cycle one was initiated by the first author and explored the bullying definition at the school and how this was understood by the school community. Online questionnaires and a focus group were used to collect data. Decisions around data collection methods, including where and when to collect the data as well as the dissemination process, were decided on by the research team together. Cycle two was initiated by the research team, following analysis of cycle one data. This second cycle explored an issue of importance to the students of the school: that of the 'snitch' and how participants conceptualised 'serious' and 'not serious' bullying. Paper questionnaires and student-led interviews were used to collect data. Cycle three focussed on the tangible 'action' from the project: the development of a draft anti-bullying strategy for the school. R4U members included Taha, Hanik, Patrick, Amy and Hope.[2] At each stage of the project, training was provided to the young researchers as detailed in the following.

As the project evolved, the use of evaluation enabled us to ascertain how R4U interpreted their own participation and to subsequently make changes to enhance this experience as necessary. Percy-Smith and Karen Malone (2001) argue that participatory opportunities should be *inclusive*, meaning that changes are made within the system to accommodate the participation of children, rather than *integrated*, which means, they argue, expecting children to participate in predefined ways and structures (*italics* in original text). The three evaluations started from the premise that participation was already happening (Moules and O'Brien 2012). They took place at 6 months, 18 months and 36 months to assess the perceived level of participation of each research team member and to address any potential issues before progressing with the project. The decision to conduct these evaluations was made by the first author.

Evaluating participation

Evaluation one

Evaluation one was conducted approximately halfway through cycle one. This cycle involved a questionnaire given to all students, parents and school staff and a focus group with students. By this point, the research team had received some training, participated in the ethical approval process, decided the data collection methods and carried out the pilot study. R4U members were asked to plot their own participation along a continuum ranging from full involvement on the left to no involvement on the right. A series of questions on how they viewed their own participation were asked, and reflective dialogue enabled discussion of the participatory process. Questions focussed on the decision-making process around data collection methods and involvement in conducting the research overall up to this point.

A theme evident in this short evaluation was that if R4U members were not attending all meetings and present when decisions were made, they regarded this as non-involvement. It was important, therefore, for the first author and R4U to revisit what participation meant to the team and what was expected from everybody while involved in the project. Alice McIntyre (2008) suggests that quality rather than quantity in terms of the number of meetings attended is what is important in participatory research. The research team took this stance and agreed that it was crucial for the project, and indeed their own satisfaction, that team members participated on their own terms and acknowledged that there would be times when not everybody could attend meetings.

It was clear when unanimous group decisions were made, such as in the development of the questionnaire. The first author provided R4U with a sample questionnaire developed by another group of young people she was working with at this time. R4U did not like this format: 'It's very long' (Hanik).

A decision was made by the group to keep our questionnaire succinct and to the point: 'We don't want to ask them about things that aren't related to our topic. I think this questionnaire asks way too many things' (Patrick).

R4U members were clear that they wanted a 'to the point' questionnaire. They were certain that students would not complete the questionnaire if it was long-winded. An assumption from the first author was that R4U would welcome this example because it had been designed by another group of young people and not adults, but this was not the case. This reiterated that a tool designed by one group of young people would not necessarily be chosen by another group of young people. Furthermore, this process showed that R4U felt able to express their concerns about the methods we were using rather than accepting a format because it was presented to them by an adult. The questionnaire used for data collection was designed by the research team together, specifically for this project.

There were also times when some decisions did not suit all group members. For example, Taha was adamant that he did not like asking participants about their ethnic origin on the questionnaire: 'I absolutely hate this question!' (Taha). Collating demographic data, such as age, gender and ethnicity, is typical of research conducted in the UK. In acknowledging Taha's reluctance to use this question, we discussed reasons why it might be important to the research and decided that as the school had a varied ethnic mix, the data could divulge information about bullying and the specific ethnic groups of participants. The team felt that this information could be useful to our findings while at the same time remaining sensitive to Taha's reluctance to use the question. We talked about the best way to frame this question, and Sarah (an earlier young researcher who left the team) suggested, 'Why don't we use the list the school uses?' The team agreed. Taha would have preferred if we did not ask the question at all. In fact, our data did not show any findings specifically related to any ethnic group in either of the data collection cycles. Furthermore, a number of participants from cycle two did not answer the question about ethnic origin.

These examples and others highlight what Perpetua Kirby *et al.* (2003) suggest about participation being about having some influence over decisions and actions and not merely about being present or taking part. R4U understanding that their individual roles in the project were valued was of paramount importance. Equally, it was important that they understood that decisions were made to enhance the rigour and trustworthiness of the study, despite agreement not being sought by all members of the team. O'Kane (2008) reiterates that when young people are given space to participate on their own terms, they can be more involved in meetings and are further motivated to take an active role in other aspects of the research. Consequently, this short evaluation highlighted the importance of providing meaningful opportunities for R4U to be involved in decision-making and in *aspects* of decision-making.

Evaluation one concluded that participation in decision-making and actions is more than just the end result. Decision-making includes a process of generating ideas, discussing the ideas and reaching a decision on what to do together. It also includes having the freedom to suggest ideas whilst being able to agree or disagree with others in a safe space. The learning taken from evaluation one into evaluation two was used to understand how R4U viewed their contribution to decision-making and how their individual contributions impacted the decisions made.

Evaluation two

Evaluation two used the Dual Axis Model of Participation (DMP) framework (Moules and O'Brien 2012) to evaluate participation 18 months into the process. By this point, we were preparing to collect data for cycle two. The DMP focusses on two dimensions of participation: *'decision making'* and *'initiation and direction'*. As a project evolves, the balance of each is either with the young researchers or the adult researcher. The model uses these two dimensions of participation and places them along two separate continuums as shown in Figure 10.1 below.

This second evaluation used this framework but focussed on *'decision-making'* and *'control and direction'* (rather than initiation and direction), and in taking evaluation one's conclusions into account, it recognised who has the *'ideas'* as a further dimension. Six questions about the process were asked to date, and R4U members were instructed to plot their perceived levels of participation along the three continuums for each question. All questions asked R4U to consider where they saw the balance of power as 'adult-led', 'young person-led' or 'shared' in relation to aspects of the process, such as data collection activities, data analysis and others.

Once all R4U members had plotted their individual perceptions of participation, a dialogical exchange took place. It was clear that participation was construed differently for each person. Taha, for example, was consistent in his interpretation. For the most part, he believed that *decisions* and *ideas*

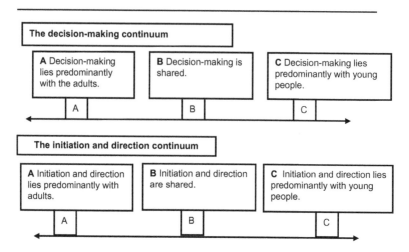

Figure 10.1 Two dimensions of participation.
Source: (Moules and O'Brien 2012).

rested with R4U, while the adult *controlled* and *directed* the activities: 'I felt I had an equal influence throughout all parts' (Taha).

Hanik, on the other hand, suggested that most activities were shared between R4U and the adult or led by R4U: 'Since I've been at every meeting, I understand nearly all the aspects' (Hanik).

Amy and Hope felt more involved at various stages of the project: '... how data was arranged and the focus groups and expressing my opinions' (Hope). 'The focus group and the analysis' (Amy).

Patrick proposed that *'decision-making'*, *'ideas'* and *'control/direction'* changed, depending on the context of the activity: 'It depended on what we were doing and who was there' (Patrick).

The ethics and value base of this study recognised the co-construction of knowledge through human relationships and collaboration; consequently, no perception, was wrong and each viewpoint was valid. For the most part, R4U perceived that *ideas* were generated by the young researchers, while the adult took *control/direction*, and *decision-making* was shared. The *ideas* generated by R4U were crucial for data collection and analysis in terms of their insider knowledge as well as for team building and developing collegiality between themselves and the adult researcher (enjoyment through games). The first author was perceived, by R4U, as taking the lead when it was necessary, but through these dynamics, a partnership developed in which power and participation levels varied and changed all the time. This perception of participation as changing and moving from task to task has been identified previously by others, such as in Jonathan Quetzal Tritter and Alison McCallum's (2006) 'mosaic' and Shirley White *et al.*'s (1994) 'kaleidoscope'.

A power shift was observed in deciding the research topic for cycle two, not only between the adult and the young researchers but also *between* the young researchers themselves. Patrick, for example, observed Hanik and Taha as being the *decision-makers* as opposed to either the adult or the young people as a collective. Ruth Sinclair (2004) acknowledges the power imbalances between children and adults in any participatory activity, while Moules and O'Brien (2012) propose that power can be shared. Evaluation two shows that not all of the power rested with adults, nor did it rest with R4U, but power was shared between adults and children. Similar to Moules and O'Brien (2012), this evaluation recognised participation as fluid, a situation in which a partnership can develop between adults and children as they move through the participatory process. This is a contrast to the linear models of participation, which suggest that participation is fully achieved once children are leading the projects.

It was imperative for this project that attention be afforded to what the students of the school were telling us through the research. However, it was also important to understand how R4U perceived their own participation and being afforded opportunities to vocalise any concerns or changes they would like to make. Of particular interest to R4U was using more games in their training: 'Sometimes it's boring just doing loads of school stuff, we need more activities' (Hope).

This request led to games being reintroduced as learning tools for cycle two, which empowered R4U to learn through fun and participate on their own terms, not an adult-led agenda (Randall 2012, Raffety 2015, Percy-Smith 2015). The use of games or arts-based approaches, argues Duncan Randall (2012), encourages adults to join children in play rather than consider methodological advantages. These approaches can add to the development of relationships and trust between adults and children (Randall 2012).

Evaluations one and two focussed on the participation of the young researchers and, in line with a PAR framework, allowed for planning, acting, observing and reflecting. Consequently, changes were made to the research to enhance the experiences for R4U. However, it was important that the role of the adult researcher was not overlooked as Mannion (2007, p. 414) proposes, '…a research agenda dedicated to listening to children's voices alone will not suffice to help us understand these processes which are as much about adults as they are about children.'

The process enabled the first author to consider the various dimensions of participation in this project. Based on evaluation two, three conclusions were drawn:

1   Different perceptions of participation for all team members were observed;
2   An obvious power shift occurred, not only from adult to young person but between young people;
3   The use of the continuums enabled dialogue about how participation was happening.

Evaluation three

The third and final evaluation rested on the adult interpretation of the participatory process. The first author used the continuum concept from evaluation two and plotted her own interpretation of participation across the lifespan of the project.

It was the interpretation of the first author that there were times when she led with *ideas, decision-making* and *direction*, while at other times R4U, took the lead, and equally, there were times when these activities were shared. The first author discussed her interpretations with R4U; for the most part, they agreed, but in some cases, they disagreed: 'I think it's perfect – with the ethics though, I think that was more you telling us. More related to you than with us in terms of what you had to do' [an application to university ethics committee] (Taha).

Hanik proposed that the first author had more input than she suggested: 'I think the interviews weren't entirely us but you as well' (Hanik).

Meanwhile, Amy noticed a situation in which R4U had had more input than the first author suggested: 'I agree with that but I also think the first focus group was half and half not just you' (Amy).

R4U felt able to disagree with the first author about her interpretations. Indeed, knowledge contribution from R4U and the first author moved back and forth along the continuum from adult-led, young person-led and shared, depending on the context of the activity. Adult-led knowledge was particularly evident at the beginning of the project, when training was delivered, and in the first author's leading the decision on which methods to use for data collection and analysis. For example, in the early months of this project, the first author perceived that much of the *control* and the *ideas* rested with her in providing training and ensuring that all team members were happy with the process. Nonetheless, from the outset, R4U were actively involved in making decisions. We made early decisions together about times and number of meetings as well as how we would begin to collect data.

There were times when it was necessary for the first author to take control of the decision-making processes; an example can be seen in the following of university procedures when seeking ethical approval. Fox (2013) critiques the process of ethical approval when engaging in participatory research. She argues that ethical guidelines are usually unfamiliar with the theoretical underpinnings of children being viewed as social actors and therefore rarely allow topic guides to be developed in conjunction with young researchers as the process develops. Typically, ethics panels prefer topic guides and other tools to be developed by adults prior to the research commencing (Fox 2013). This was not the experience during this project. At the beginning of each cycle, an ethics application was submitted to the university ethics panel, but as our tools were not fully developed, we were granted permission to submit them once they had been finalised, and ethics approval was then granted on chair's action. In cycle one, R4U were informed about the ethics process, but they were equally happy for the first author to take the lead. In cycle two, this changed somewhat as R4U had a greater understanding of the ethical approval process and therefore contributed to the application.

The first author perceived that the *ideas* about data analysis in cycle one were adult-led. Her role in interpreting and analysing the data was in enabling the team to capture what participants were saying as a collective but also to ensure that individual stories were not lost. The data analysis activities in cycle one acted as training exercises for R4U, with the intention that they would be further involved in analysing the data in cycle two. R4U, on the other hand, viewed the data analysis activities in cycles one and two as predominantly shared. It is interesting that R4U viewed the power imbalances differently than the first author, but this may be a result of the reciprocal relationship between young people and adults not being viewed as the norm for this group of young researchers. In fact, in an unpublished paper written by the research team, R4U stated, 'We hope that researchers in the future will take Niamh's example and provide students with their own opportunity to carry out their own research'.

The shift from conducting the research from an adult standpoint at the outset and moving towards a collegial partnership with R4U, based on what the data and dialogue in the research team was showing, moved the power dimensions in this project. Martin Woodhead and Dorothy Faulkner (2008) remind us that all too often, data, such as interview transcripts, are analysed based on adult assumptions and ideologies. In this project, however, the voice of the child was central, not only to collecting the data but also in the analysis. The use of insider knowledge enabled R4U to interpret the data in a different way to the first author as they understood the contextual environment and the bullying situation in the school. Through the process of PAR the research team were able to construct meaning together, based not entirely on our own assumptions and ideologies but also from the viewpoint of the research participants (Thomson and Gunter 2009).

An important element of the participatory process is providing multiple opportunities for young researchers to be actively involved in decision-making. Furthermore relationship-building and realising the role played by adults in the process are equally important. Evaluation three allowed for reflection on the adult role in the participatory process and, through our dialogical exchanges, enabled the young researchers to revisit how participation happened for them during the project as a whole. It became apparent to the first author that providing opportunities for R4U to make decisions without adults was not the aim of this project – the aim was to develop collegial relationships with these young people so that together, we could generate knowledge that was paramount. This meant that the adult role needed to be acknowledged in the process as equally important. Mannion (2007) discusses the relationships between adults and children in which the adult cannot be 'cut out' in terms of how young people participate.

Discussion

The three evaluations showed participation to be varied and complex. Within the confines of this project, participation was observed as being characteristic of the following:

1   Decision-making is more than the end result;
2   The adult plays an active role in the process;
3   Young people have an active and valid contribution to make as researchers.

Decision-making is more than the end result

Evaluation one concluded that R4U did not perceive their role in decision-making as active if they were not present when a decision was made. As the project evolved, R4U were able to recognise how their ideas, views and opinions fed into the decision-making process alongside the first author's. Furthermore, they were forthcoming with their opinions and views about how changes could be made to the research process. Due to the first author actively listening to what R4U said and providing feedback on how their input contributed to decisions, the young researchers viewed adults as willing to relinquish some of their power and work with them in a collegial way, as is evidenced in other studies (Kirby *et al.* 2003, Bragg and Fielding 2005). Furthermore, honesty with R4U and the participating students about how views, opinions and research findings were likely to impact the overall decisions made were demonstrated (Sinclair 2004). The evaluations showed how adults and children can negotiate the research space and generate knowledge through an equal working relationship whilst acknowledging the potential power issues. This was important because Fielding (2004) and Randall (2012) propose that children could decide not to participate in research if they perceive that their views will not be taken seriously or acted upon. Mannion (2009) and Randall (2012) thus suggest that the way that adults communicate to children that they value their input will have an impact on how the findings from participatory research are understood. This also has an impact on the quality of the relationships between adults and young researchers.

The adult plays an active role in the process

Research recommends that adults should consider how research spaces, and spaces for children more generally, are co-constructed by the actions of the adults who work with children and young people (Fielding 2004, Mannion 2007). These relationships are key for determining which children get heard, what ideas children can talk about and what differences this process will make to the adult-child relationship (Mannion 2007, Fitzgerald *et al.* 2009).

In this project, the research team relied on adults in many ways. First, R4U relied on the first author to initially facilitate the participatory process and guide the research. Second, the full team were reliant on other adults, in the form of parents and staff, to participate in data collection and on adult gate-keepers, in the form of school authorities. Relationships between adults and young people were tested on numerous occasions. In cycle one, the questionnaire was sent to parents and teachers, but many adults chose not to complete it. This left team members despondent as gaps were evident in our data. We wanted to ensure that we captured the viewpoints of all stakeholders because the research team wanted to hear adult views too, recognising these as important alongside students' views. This recognition enabled the research team to encourage adult participation in cycle two whilst respecting the wishes of adults who chose not to participate. In essence, a role reversal was noted as young people were implementing measures, so adults could participate on their own terms.

Mannion (2007) and Erin L. Raffety (2015) consider children researching children. They propose that just because children are involved in conducting their own research, the process might not necessarily expand children's participation and autonomy nor might this process address power differentials between adults and children. Raffety (2015) discusses researchers' acknowledgements of the social differences between adult researchers and children in the research field. These differences were acknowledged from the outset: The first author was an adult working with young people and therefore was perceived as an authority figure. In the beginning, R4U insisted on calling her 'Mrs O'Brien' rather than 'Niamh'. She explained to them that she was not there in a teaching capacity but to conduct this research in partnership with them. Calling her 'Mrs O'Brien' put her in charge, so they reluctantly agreed to call her 'Niamh'. It was obvious that some members were initially uncomfortable with this as Hanik stated when referring to the school authorities: 'They won't be happy here with us not addressing you as Mrs' (Hanik).

By the end of the project, the perception that R4U had of the first author in a teacher role had changed. At one meeting towards the end of the project, we discussed how the role she had in the research team might be considered alongside that of a teacher: 'It's not like you're a teacher because you're learning from us and we're learning from you. With teachers it's just one way' (Hanik).

Furthermore, R4U reflected on their role as active researchers in the project and considered the value of peer-led interviews without adults present: 'There were some things they [student participants] would tell us and not adults because we are closer in age' (Amy). 'They feel more comfortable like they're not getting anyone else into trouble' (Patrick).

Through this process of ongoing reflection and evaluation, the team were able to see how their viewpoints and ideas were feeding into the whole research process, and they were participating on their own terms, not those decided by adults (Randall 2012, Raffety 2015, Percy-Smith 2015). Indeed, R4U began to understand the unique role that all team members had in the project. Fielding (2004) and Mannion (2009) acknowledge that the relationship between adult and young researchers are interdependent and can blossom as both adults and young people understand each other's unique roles. Taha recognised this notion and likened the team to a cricket team:

> It's like we're a cricket team with 11 players and the coach. The coach helps and supports the team but the team plays the game. Everyone has to work together if you want to win the game. You're like the coach and we're like the team.
>
> (Taha)

Indeed, the literature recognises that a limitation of childhood research is the reliance that young people have on adults to work with them and facilitate change (Kellett 2010). However, as the project progressed, R4U perceived the role of the adult in a different way – not as a facilitator or teacher but as a team member with an equal contribution to make – thus minimising the social differences between adult and young people (Randall 2012, Raffety 2015).

Young people have an active and valid contribution to make as researchers

Although the benefits of involving children in participatory activities are recognised in the literature (Kellett 2010), Percy-Smith (2015, p. 3) suggests that these changes have had limited impact 'on the position of children and young people in society'. A key aspect of this project was the development of an action that would continue the work of the project once the research had ended, and this was seen in the development of a draft anti-bullying strategy that was accepted by the school. Such initiatives show how the work continues after the research has ended (O'Brien 2014).

The training provided to R4U was tailored to the needs of this project, and Kellett (2010) suggests that generic in-depth research training provided to children, which they can draw upon to initiate their own projects, shifts the power imbalance towards children. In this case, children are leading their own projects with support from adults, but adults are not managing the research. This shift in power was evident in evaluation two in the process of decision-making and again in evaluation three, when R4U members disagreed with the first author about her interpretation of where the participation happened. The contribution made by R4U in terms of their unique insider knowledge added to the depth of the findings, in which we captured a collective picture of the bullying issues in the school but at the same time encapsulated individual unique stories from each of our participants.

Conclusion

Combining findings from the three evaluations highlighted that decision-making and participation is more than the end result but is a process of generating ideas, discussing these ideas and having the freedom to agree and disagree with others in a safe space. An initial aim of the project was ultimately for the decision-making to be led by R4U, with the adult facilitating the process. However, a process of reciprocity ensued that saw the development of a relationship between the adult and R4U in conducting the research together and developing a tangible 'action' in the form of an anti-bullying strategy for the school. It was evident that R4U had a wealth of knowledge to contribute as 'insiders', and without this knowledge, the findings and action generated would not have been the same.

Throughout this study, every effort was made to share control and power over the process, including over data interpretation. That power can be shared was evident across the evaluations, but there were times when the power was in favour of the adult and times when power was in favour of the young researchers, depending on the context of the research activity. The use of constant evaluation encouraged a redress of power and enabled both adult and young researchers to critically reflect on the process as the project evolved.

Notes

1 The term 'children and young people', 'child' and 'young person' will be used interchangeably throughout this chapter. These terms are understood as referring to any person under 18 years of age.
2 These are the real names of the young researchers as they requested I use them rather than pseudonyms.

References

Bragg, S., and Fielding, M., 2005. It's an equal thing... It's about achieving together: Student voices and the possibility of a radical collegiality. In: H. Street, and J. Temperley (eds.) *Improving schools through collaborative enquiry.* London: Continuum, 105–135.

Davey, C., 2010. Children's Participation in Decision making. A Summary Report on Progress made up to 2010. Available from: http://www.participationworks.org. uk/files/webfm/files/npf~/npf_publications/A%20Summary%20Report_jun10. pdf [Accessed 13th January 2014].

Fielding, M., 2004. Transformative approaches to student voice: Theoretical underpinnings, recalcitrant realities. *British Educational Research Journal*, 30 (2), 295–311.

Fitzgerald, R., Graham, A., Smith, A., and Taylor, N., 2009. Children's participation as a struggle over recognition: Exploring the promise of dialogue. In: B. Percy-Smith, and N. Thomas (eds.) *A handbook of children and young people's participation: Perspectives from theory and practice.* London: Routledge, Taylor and Francis Group, 293–305.

Fox, R., 2013. Resisting participation: Critiquing participatory research methodologies with young people. *Journal of Youth Studies*, 16 (8), 986–999.

Hinton, R., 2008. Children's participation and good governance: Limitations of the theoretical literature. *International Journal of Children's Rights*, 16, 285–300.

James, A., 2007. Giving voice to children's voices: Practices and problems, pitfalls and potentials. *American Anthropologist*, 109 (2), 261–272.

Kellett, M., 2010. Small shoes, big steps! Empowering children as active researchers. *American Journal of Community Psychology*, 46, 195–203.

Kellett, M., Forrest, R., Dent, N., and Ward, S., 2004. 'Just teach us the skills please, we'll do the rest': Empowering ten-year-olds as active researchers. *Children and Society*, 18, 329–343.

Kemmis, S., and McTaggart, R., 1988. *The Action Research Planner*, 3rd ed. Victoria: Deakin University Press.

Kirby, P., Lanyon, C., Cronin, K., and Sinclair, R., 2003. *Building a Culture of Participation: Involving Children and Young People in Policy, Service Planning, Delivery and Evaluation: Handbook*. London: Department for Education and Skills, [online]. Available from: http://core.ac.uk/download/pdf/9983740.pdf [Accessed 10th February 2015].

Mannion, G., 2007. Going spatial, going relational: why "listening to children" and children's participation needs reframing. *Discourse: Studies in the Cultural Politics of Education*, 28 (3), 405–420.

Mannion, G., 2009. After participation: The socio-spatial performance of intergenerational becoming. In: B. Percy-Smith, and N. Thomas (eds.) *A handbook of children and young people's participation: Perspectives from theory and practice*. London: Routledge, Taylor and Francis Group, 330–342.

McIntyre, A., 2008. *Participatory Action Research. Qualitative Research Methods*, Series 52. Thousand Oaks, CA: A Sage University Paper.

Moules, T., and O'Brien, N., 2012. Participation in perspective: Reflections from research projects. *Nurse Researcher*, 19 (2), 17–22.

O'Brien, N., 2014. "I didn't want to be known as a snitch": Using PAR to explore bullying in a private day and boarding school. *Childhood Remixed*. Conference Edition, February 2014, 86–96.

O'Brien, N., and Moules, T., 2007. So round the spiral again: A reflective participatory research project with children and young people. *Educational Action Research Journal*, 15 (3), 385–402.

O'Brien, N., and Moules, T., 2013. Not sticks and stones but tweets and texts: Findings from a national cyberbullying project. *Pastoral Care in Education*, 31 (1), 53–66.

O'Brien, N., Munn-Giddings, C., and Moules, T., 2017/8. The repercussions of reporting bullying: Some experiences of students at secondary school. *Pastoral Care in Education*, accepted.

O'Kane, C., 2008. The development of participatory techniques: Facilitating children's views about decisions which affect them. In: P. Christensen, and A. James (eds.) 2nd ed. *Research with children: Perspectives and practices*. Oxon: Routledge, 125–155.

Percy-Smith, B., 2015. Negotiating active citizenship: Young people's participation in everyday spaces. In: K. P. Kallio, and S. Mills (eds.) *Politics, citizenship and rights. geographies of children and young people* (7). London: Springer. [online]. Available from: http://eprints.hud.ac.uk/23226/1/Geogs_of_youth_citizenship_Dec18_revised.pdf [Accessed 13th March 2015].

Percy-Smith, B., and Malone, K., 2001. Making children's participation in neighbourhood settings relevant to the everyday lives of young people. *PLA notes*, 42, 18–22.

Raffety, E. L., 2015. Minimizing social distance: Participatory research with children. *Childhood*, 22 (3), 409–422.

Randall, D., 2012. Revisiting Mandell's 'least adult' role and engaging with children's voices in research. *Nurse Researcher*, 19 (3), 39–43.

Sinclair, R., 2004. Participation in practice: Making it meaningful, effective and sustainable. *Children and Society*, 18 (2), 106–118.

Stoudt, B. G., 2009. The role of language & discourse in the investigation of privilege: Using participatory action research to discuss theory. Develop methodology & interrupt power. *Urban Review*, 41, 7–28.

Thomson, P., and Gunter, H., 2009. Students' participation in school change: Action research on the ground. In: S. Noffke, and B. Somekh (eds.) *The SAGE handbook of educational action research*. London: Sage, 409–419.

Tritter, J. Q., and McCallum, A., 2006. The snakes and ladders of user involvement: Moving beyond Arnstein. *Health Policy*, 76 (2), 156–168.

White, S. A., Sadanandan, N. K., and Ashcroft, J., 1994. *Participatory Communication: Working for Change and Development*. New Delhi: Sage Publications.

Winter, R., and Munn-Giddings, C., 2001. *A Handbook for Action Research in Health and Social Care*. London: Routledge.

Woodhead, M., and Faulkner, D., 2008. Subjects, objects or participants? Dilemmas of psychological research with children. In: P. Christensen, and A. James (eds.) 2nd ed. *Research with children: Perspectives and practices*. Oxon: Routledge, 10–39.

Reciprocal social work and social policy
Conclusions

In his last diary 'Smiling in Slow Motion', the late film director and gay activist Derek Jarman (2001, p. 43) reflects on politics in general and admonishes some of his peers for assuming and colluding with the view that 'steps forward' always occur through top-down parliamentary legislation. This, he comments,

> ...is a mistake, steps forward come by the example in our lives...the aim is to open up discourse and with it broader horizons...

What did he mean by this? No doubt many things, but in relation to the themes threaded through the chapters in this book, there is an important message about the everyday relationships we forge and the ways in which we behave to one another, both informally, as citizens in our communities, and formally, in welfare organisations. The ways in which we develop and conduct these relationships can either reinforce or collude with existing inequalities and power imbalances. Alternatively, those social relations can embody a challenge to existing understandings and practices. Developing an approach that we are calling a *reciprocal social work and social policy* is one way in which we offer an alternative to current neoliberal and individualistic approaches.

At the heart of the approach is an emphasis on social relations, which are crucial to our well-being and central to making our lives meaningful or otherwise. There is a robust research knowledge base that illustrates how social relations are accessed differently in different populations but how they consistently have an important and significant influence on health and well-being (see Antonucci *et al.* 2014, p. 83; see also authors in this book). However, it is not enough to be in a social relationship; it is also the quality and form of these relations that matters. If relationships do not last or do not support the well-being of individuals, they can be viewed as one-sided or abusive. Reciprocal relations are based on mutual understanding, respect and trust, which create a sense of equality between different partners. They give a person the feeling that they are respected as a person and do not need to pretend to be someone else.

We have deliberately steered clear of one overarching definition of reciprocity in the book but rather have offered readers a wide interpretation from authors working in different welfare fields and in different cultural contexts. Authors in this book have variously defined 'reciprocity' in relation to philosophy, method and experience. Whilst their definitions are context-specific and drawn from a range of different theorists (such as Becker 1990, Bourdieu 1990, Fiske 1992, Gouldner 1960, Kolm 2008, Sen 2009), there are common themes that run through their discussions:

- Interdependence in relationships, in which people are able to both give and receive support;
- Recognising that people have different things to offer in this mutual exchange, based on their strengths, and acknowledging their vulnerabilities; i.e. an exchange can be both material and immaterial; people can give and take in different forms;
- The quality of relationships that are both egalitarian and mutual, in which all parties are treated fairly and feel listened to and 'heard'
- Reciprocal experiences that are strongly associated with feelings of empathy, satisfaction and even love.

Various mechanisms, attitudes and approaches are identified as critical to the process of building reciprocal relationships, such as trust, humour, co-learning, respect, openness, sympathy and goodwill as well as the conscious creation of spaces for the renegotiation and reshaping of conventional practices. Enablers of these mechanisms are illustrated in different ways throughout the book and include reflective practices, both in professional work and research practices that involve all parties, and the identification of and learning gained from citizens and service-users' own reciprocal practices and networks, which support each other in the community, involving service-users in processes to co-produce social work knowledge that informs policies and practices. Working practices that offer more scope for the traditional practitioner and service-user relationships to be reframed are more likely to engender a reciprocal relationship: for example, the use of group and community-based services and collaborative methods in research, education and practice. Respecting the different but complementary roles of experiential and professional knowledge is at the heart of enabling policies and practices.

The chapters of this book illuminate citizens' reciprocal actions with each other as embedded both in everyday life activities and in different institutionalised practices linked to social work. However, because people and the systems they create do not always support reciprocal relations – for instance, in forms of corruption or nepotism – there is a need for societal rules that are negotiated by democratic regulations and democratic decision-making based on an understanding of social rights and equalities. That is why both social work and social policy are needed to help promote equality between citizens in the societies that can support their well-being and create a just social and health service system. Reciprocity, when it is understood positively, is like an ideal type or aim for collectiveness or togetherness in a society. It can also work as a societal goal for social work and social policy and its practice, which is negotiated through political decision-making in certain places and times.

Reciprocity is a particularly important and interesting concept in the context of asymmetrical and hierarchical relationships, such as professional-service-user, interviewer-interviewee, student-educator and child-adult relationships. All of these come along with an unequal distribution of power that needs to be critically scrutinised when achieving reciprocal practices and policies aiming to enhance the well-being of individuals. Reciprocal practices focus on processes that flow two ways, which is an immediate challenge to the hierarchical order of a variety of formal and informal relationships relevant to social work. Reciprocity seems to be particularly important for people who are dependent upon others and are often described as those who 'receive' rather than 'give'. In this book, we have seen various authors outline the ways in which discourses (and, indeed, policies and practices) related to 'risk' can provide a barrier to achieving equality in relationships. Unfortunately, in public discourse, needing help is often described and experienced as shameful and stigmatising. In addition, prevalent discourses on 'scrounging', 'parasitism' and 'burdens' cast social actors in unhelpful relationships with and to one another.

Is it possible to increase reciprocity in professional or formal relationships? Service-users of social work might say that they are not heard. People can feel as if the professional is only taking care of their duties rather than also caring for them and listening to them as another human being. Understanding the nature of reciprocity offers social work and social policy possibilities to see how inequalities or social problems are generated in a community setting – for instance, in mutual, intergenerational or even professional relationships. This understanding may create a good basis for acknowledging that difficulties are often community-based, not just individual. If social work professionalism and social policy practice are developed reciprocally, they require at least two different kinds of change in their professional approaches.

First, there is a need to further develop the equality between professionals and service-users in mutual encounters. When reciprocity is based on a sense of equality, people are helped on their own terms. This kind of professionalism requires professionals to engage with service-users and work with them to solve life challenges rather than viewing them from a fixed professional position. Even in challenging situations that require the social worker to prioritise the rights of someone who is vulnerable (for example, in child protection), it is still important that understanding is shown to the service-user. There is a sense that both parties can learn from each other and feel and show empathy or sympathy, which generates respect, interest and trust in others. When a professional relationship is reciprocal, it is empowering, both for the professionals and the service-users. Both have a feeling that they are valued as persons with their own knowledge and experiences. They have a feeling that they are making decisions together, respecting both parties. There may not always be an agreement of opinions, but there is a possibility to feel understood.

Second, in terms of understanding the collective nature of reciprocity, there is an urgent need for community-based services and methods that value people's own capacities to solve problems and find solutions to them. Sometimes, individual support is enough, but often, the nature of difficulties is community-based, for instance, in loneliness or bullying. In these situations, there should be more ways to support the individual in their communities and work with communities recognising common similar life experiences. In this way, people can get a feeling that they are not alone with their difficulties and can share their experiences or interests. Creating these kinds of helping and supporting communities is not only a question of social or health services – it has implications for inter-professional, whole community planning, including, for instance, use in workplaces, schools, day care, elderly care and housing that respects, supports and builds on citizens' own social networks and commitments. This understanding demands the development of services and professional work that respects people's own wishes and resources and the exploration ways of working with people and their communities.

As we have seen throughout the book, reciprocity is a fundamental human philosophy and practice that takes different forms in different historical periods and cultural settings. It is a concept at the heart of a philosophical framework and is expressed in shared action and trust between individuals and their communities in a variety of forms. It is both 'common' and 'profound'. Reciprocity is profound in the sense that practiced positively, it enhances the equality and well-being of people. It draws on the resources and skills of people, foregrounding their strengths and acknowledging their vulnerabilities. It offers a vision that promotes interdependence, mutual respect and co-learning and moves us away from individualistic models of health and social care to a collective vision that understands and locates people in their various networks (family, friends, peers and geographic and interest communities). It endorses models of policy and practice that work with strengths and resources, not only of individual clients but also of collectives. Practices that begin from the standpoint of enablement and mutual respect lead to a variety of enabling roles that usefully support, rather than undermine, people's own agency and resources.

The chapters of this book emphasise that everyone has something to give and that being able to reciprocate – as well as behave respectfully – is essential for one's well-being and self-esteem. The chapters also raise the need for future qualitative and quantitative research into reciprocity focussing on experiences of bidirectionality, receiving and giving within welfare services, and social work and society at large as ways of challenging existing hierarchical power relationships. The theme of the book also calls for the use of collaborative and creative methods in practice, research and education as well as the co-production of professional and experiential knowledge and mutual learning.

References

Antonucci, T. C., Ajrouch, K. J., and Birditt, K. S., 2014. The Convoy Model: Explaining Social Relations from a Multidisciplinary Perspective. Special Issue: Remembering Our Roots. *The Gerontologists*, 54, (1), 82–92.

Becker, L. C., 1990. *Reciprocity*. London: Routledge & Kegan Paul.

Bourdieu, P., 1990. *In Other Words*. Stanford: Stanford University Press.

Fiske, A. P., 1992. The Four Elementary Forms of Sociality: Framework for a Unified Theory of Social Relations. *Psychological Review*, 99 (4), 689–723.

Gouldner, A. W., 1960. The Norm of Reciprocity: A Preliminary Statement. *American Sociological Review*, 25 (2), 161–178.

Jarman, D., 2001. *Smiling in Slow Motion*. London: Vintage.

Kolm, S. E., 2008. *Reciprocity. An Economics of Social Relations*. Cambridge: Cambridge University Press.

Sen, A., 2009. *The Idea of Justice*. London: Penguin Books.